SPRINGHOUSE

Professional Care Guide

Psychiatric Disorders

SPRINGHOUSE

Professional Care Guide

Psychiatric Disorders

Springhouse Corporation
Springhouse, Pennsylvania

Staff

Senior Publisher
Matthew Cahill

Clinical Manager
Cindy Tryniszewski, RN, MSN

Art Director
John Hubbard

Senior Editor
June Norris

Editors
Edith McMahon, Elizabeth Weinstein

Clinical Editors
Judith Schilling McCann, RN, BSN; Beverly Tscheschlog, RN

Designers
Stephanie Peters (senior associate art director), Lynn Foulk (book designer)

Copy Editors
Cynthia C. Breuninger (manager), Lynette High, Doris Weinstock, Lewis Adams, Nancy Papsin

Typography
Diane Paluba (manager), Elizabeth Bergman, Joyce Rossi Biletz, Phyllis Marron, Robin Mayer, Valerie Rosenberger

Manufacturing
Deborah C. Meiris (director), Pat Dorshaw, T.A. Landis

Production Coordination
Patricia McCloskey

Editorial Assistants
Beverly Lane, Mary Madden, Dianne Tolbert

The cover illustration depicts the transmission of dopamine, a neurotransmitter, across a nerve ending synapse. Altered dopamine levels in the brain may be linked to psychiatric disorders, such as schizophrenia. Illustration by Kevin A. Somerville.

A member of the Reed Elsevier plc group

PCG4-010395

Library of Congress Cataloging-in-Publication Data
Psychiatric disorders.
    p. cm. – (Professional care guides)
Includes bibliographical references and index.
1. Psychiatric nursing. 2. Psychology, Pathological.
    I. Springhouse Corporation. II. Series.
    [DNLM: 1. Mental Disorders.
    WM 100 P97343 1995]
RC440.P733 1995
610.73′68 – dc20
DNLM/DLC   94-33379
ISBN: 0-87434-781-5   CIP

Contents

Contributors and Consultants

Marlene Ciranowicz, RN, MSN, CDE
Independent Nurse Consultant
Dresher, Pa.

Brian B. Doyle, MD
Director, Anxiety Disorders Program
Department of Psychiatry
Georgetown University Medical School
Washington, D.C.

Julie Gerhart, RPh
Long-Term Care Division
Hunsicker's Pharmacy, Inc.
Souderton, Pa.

Karen A. Jantzi, RN, MSN
Psychiatric Coordinator
Indian Creek Foundation
Harleysville, Pa.

Judith E. Meissner, RN, MSN
Nursing and Educational Consultant
Warminster, Pa.

Foreword

Few patients present as many challenges to health care professionals as those with psychiatric illnesses. And few areas of modern medicine have demonstrated as many dramatic and effective advances as has psychiatric care. At the same time, social and economic forces have propelled many psychiatric patients out of inpatient, chronic-care settings and into outpatient or short-term care settings. As a result, these patients are seeking help in greater numbers in general medical settings, and the need for nonpsychiatric clinicians to understand and treat them is increasing steadily.

Current estimates point out that one in three Americans is or will be mentally ill or directly affected by someone who is. As a result, a greater understanding of psychiatric illness becomes not only a personal concern but also a professional necessity. Supplying this understanding is the mission of *Psychiatric Disorders*. In this concise, well-written, and timely volume from the Professional Care Guide series, you'll find clear descriptions of psychiatric disorders, up-to-date summaries of diagnoses and treatments, and scores of practical suggestions for dealing with psychiatric patients.

Today, accurate diagnosis of a psychiatric disorder requires evaluating the patient on multiple axes presented in the standard, updated version of the *Diagnostic and Statistical Manual of Mental Disorders*, 4th edition *(DSM-IV)*. For ease of use, the psychiatric disorders discussed in this book parallel the order of their appearance in *DSM-IV*.

Today, psychiatric treatments are more specific and efficacious than ever before. For instance, new drugs can alleviate symptoms in even the most severe psychiatric illness, schizophrenia, with fewer adverse effects. Several new antianxiety and antidepressant drugs provide greater relief with less discomfort. New uses have been discovered for existing drugs; for example, some antidepressants also help patients with anxiety disorders. *Psychiatric Disorders* discusses these current treatments in detail.

For many health care professionals, the most valuable feature of *Psychiatric Disorders* may be its specific recommendations for what to say to psychiatric patients— and what to do. Certainly, the volatile emotions and unusual behavior of psychiatric patients challenge not only nursing and medical staff but also allied health caregivers. The interventions suggested in this book will help you better understand and deal more effectively with psychiatric patients.

Psychiatric Disorders opens with a chapter explaining the classification of psychiatric illnesses and how to perform a psychiatric evaluation. Subsequent chapters discuss disorders of infancy, childhood, and adolescence, such as mental retardation and attention-deficit hyperactivity disorder. Next follow chapters on alcohol and drug abuse and dependence, schizophrenia, and mood, anxiety, somatoform, dissociative, personality, and eating disorders.

For convenience, each disorder in the book's nine chapters is organized consistently. Each one covers causes, signs and symptoms, diagnosis, treatments, and special considerations. At the end of each chapter, you'll find a helpful self-test section. This section allows the reader to quickly evaluate understanding of the chapter's main concepts and clinical issues. Answers to these questions and the rationales appear at the back of the book.

Extensive appendices cover recommended laboratory tests during psychotropic drug therapy, drugs causing psychiatric symptoms, and schedules of controlled substances. The final appendix combines the *DSM-IV* classification with the *International Classification of Diseases,* 9th revision, *Clinical Modification.*

With its up-to-date information, clear style, and practical approach, *Psychiatric Disorders* is a must for student and practicing nurses, general practitioners, medical students, house officers, and allied health care workers.

Brian B. Doyle, MD
Director, Anxiety Disorders Program
Department of Psychiatry
Georgetown University Medical School
Washington, D.C.

CHAPTER 1

Introduction

In recent years, a convergence of social, economic, and professional forces has dramatically changed the mental health field. Community and professional organizations, for instance, have established family advocacy programs, substance abuse rehabilitation programs, stress management workshops, bereavement groups, victim assistance programs, and violence shelters. Our public education system has spread information about mental health issues. Self-help and coping books have proliferated, and media attention to mental and emotional disorders has increased.

Social changes

Today, more people than ever experience mental health problems. Some researchers blame social changes, which have altered the traditional family structure and contributed to the loss of the extended family. The result: more single parents, dysfunctional families, troubled children, and homeless people.

The loss of effective support systems strains a person's ability to cope with even minor problems. For example, a working mother may lack the necessary support to meet the demands of her job, her home, her spouse, and her children. When she views herself as ineffective in these roles, her self-esteem falters and her level of stress intensifies.

Furthermore, the incidence of teenage depression and suicide has more than tripled in the past 20 years. Alcohol and substance abuse are proliferating and their victims are becoming younger. Isolation, fear of violent crime, and loneliness have contributed to a similar rise in depression among elderly people. Combat veterans, rape victims, and child abuse victims struggle to cope with the trauma they've experienced.

Economic changes

Recent cuts in federal funding of mental health programs place future control of mental health services at the state and local level and drastically reduce the funds available for training. One result of decreased funding is increased collaboration between community psychiatric facilities (short-term inpatient, outpatient, and auxiliary services) and long-term inpatient state facilities.

Professional changes

Mental health professionals have experienced enormous changes in perspective, focus, and direction, which are reflected in the American Psychiatric Association's *Diagnostic and Statistical Manual of Mental Disorders*, 4th edition *(DSM-IV)*. With this system of classifying mental disorders, clinicians must consider many aspects of the patient's behavior, mental performance, and history, emphasizing observable data rather than subjective and theoretical impressions.

DSM-IV

The *DSM-IV* defines a mental disorder as a clinically significant behavioral or psychological syndrome or pattern that's associated with current distress (a painful symptom) or disability (impairment in one or more important areas of functioning) or with a significantly greater risk of suffering, death, pain, disability, or an important loss of freedom. This syndrome or pattern mustn't be merely an expected response such as grief over the death of a loved one. Whatever its original cause, it must currently be considered a sign of a behavioral, psychological, or biological dysfunction.

To add diagnostic detail, *DSM-IV* uses a multiaxial approach. This approach specifies that every patient be evaluated on each of the following five axes:
• *Axis I:* clinical disorder—the diagnosis (or diagnoses) that best describes the presenting complaint
• *Axis II:* personality disorders and mental retardation
• *Axis III:* general medical conditions—a description of any concurrent medical conditions or disorders
• *Axis IV:* psychosocial and environmental problems
• *Axis V:* global assessment of functioning (GAF), based on a scale of 1 to 100. The GAF scale allows evaluation of the patient's overall psychological, social, and occupational function.

The first three axes, which constitute the official diagnostic assessment, encompass the entire spectrum of mental and physical disorders. This system may require multiple diagnoses. For example, on Axis I, a patient may have both a psychoactive substance abuse disorder and a mood disorder. He may even have multiple diagnoses within the same class, as in major depression superimposed on cyclothymic disorder. A patient also may have a disorder on Axes I, II, and III simultaneously.

Axis IV documents the effect of psychosocial and environmental stressors on the patient. Examples of such stressors include marital, familial, interpersonal, occupational, domestic, financial, legal, developmental, and medical concerns as well as environmental factors and natural disasters.

Axis V measures how well the patient has functioned over the past year. It also encompasses the current level of functioning.

A patient's diagnosis after being evaluated on these five axes may look like this:
- *Axis I:* adjustment disorder with anxious mood
- *Axis II:* obsessive-compulsive personality
- *Axis III:* Crohn's disease, acute bleeding episode
- *Axis IV:* recent remarriage, death of father
- *Axis V:* GAF 65 (current).

Holistic care

An increased emphasis on holistic care has promoted a closer relationship between psychiatry and the rest of medicine. More hospitalized patients benefit from psychiatric consultations, reflecting a growing recognition of the emotional basis of physical disorders. Advances in neurobiology have revolutionized our understanding of the physiologic basis of mental function. The result: better diagnosis and treatment of mental disorders.

Psychosocial evaluation

In all clinical areas and settings, you'll encounter patients with mental and emotional problems. Begin your care of these patients with a psychosocial evaluation. For this evaluation to be effective, you need to establish a therapeutic relationship based on trust. You must communicate to the patient that his thoughts and behaviors are important. Effective communication involves both sending and receiving messages. Words count, as does nonverbal communication—eye contact, posture, facial expressions, gestures, clothing, affect, even silence. All can convey a powerful message. (See *Communication barriers,* pages 4 and 5.)

Choose a quiet, private setting for the evaluation interview. Interruptions and distractions threaten confidentiality and interfere with effective listening. If you're meeting the

Communication barriers

Ineffective communication can prevent a successful interview.

Language difficulties or differences
If the patient speaks English, try to use language that's appropriate to his educational level. Avoid medical terms that he may not understand.

If the patient speaks a foreign language or an ethnic dialect, an interpreter can help you communicate. But remember that the presence of a third person may make the patient less willing to share his feelings.

Be aware of words that can have more than one meaning. For instance, the word "bad" also can be used as slang to mean "good."

Inappropriate responses
Inadvertently, your responses to the patient can suggest disinterest, anxiety, or annoyance. Or they can imply value judgments. Examples include abruptly changing the subject or discounting the patient's feelings.

Hearing loss
If the patient can't hear you clearly, he may misinterpret your responses. If you're interviewing a patient with impaired hearing, check whether he's wearing a hearing aid. If so, is it turned on? If not, can he read lips? If possible, face him and speak clearly and slowly, using common words and keeping your questions short, simple, and direct.

If the patient is elderly, use a low tone of voice. With aging, the ability to hear high-pitched tones deteriorates first. If the patient's hearing impairment is severe, he may have to communicate by writing, or you may need to collect information from his family or friends.

Thought disorders
If the patient's thought patterns are incoherent or irrelevant, he may be unable to interpret messages correctly, focus on the interview, or provide appropriate responses.

When assessing such a patient, ask simple questions about concrete topics and clarify his responses. Encourage him to express himself clearly.

Paranoid thinking
When dealing with a paranoid patient, approach him in a nonthreatening way. Avoid touching him because he may misinterpret your touch as an attempt to harm him. Also, keep in mind that he may not mean the things he says.

Hallucinations
A hallucinating patient experiences imaginary sensory perceptions with no basis in reality. These distortions prevent him from hearing and responding appropriately.

Show concern if the patient is hallucinating, but don't reinforce his perceptions. Be as specific as possible when you give him commands. For instance, if he says he's hearing voices, tell him to stop listening to the voices and listen to you instead.

Delusions
A deluded patient defends irrational beliefs or ideas despite factual evidence to the contrary. Some delusions may be so bizarre that you'll immediately recognize them; others may be difficult to identify.

Don't condemn or agree with a patient's delusional beliefs, and don't dis-

Communication barriers *(continued)*

miss a statement because you think it's delusional. Instead, gently emphasize reality without being argumentative.

Delirium
A delirious patient experiences disorientation, hallucinations, and confusion. Misinterpretation and inappropriate responses often result.

Talk directly to such a patient and ask simple questions. Offer frequent reassurance.

Dementia
The patient who suffers dementia—an irreversible deterioration of mental capacity—may experience changes in memory and thought patterns, and his language may become distorted or slurred.

When interviewing such a patient, minimize distractions. Use simple and concise language. Avoid making any statements that could be easily misinterpreted.

patient for the first time, introduce yourself and explain the interview's purpose. Sit at a comfortable distance from the patient, and give him your undivided attention.

During the interview, adopt a professional but friendly attitude, and maintain eye contact. A calm, nonthreatening tone of voice will encourage the patient to talk more openly. Avoid value judgments. Don't rush through the interview; building a trusting therapeutic relationship takes time.

History

A patient history establishes a baseline and provides clues to the underlying or precipitating cause of the current problem. The patient may not be a reliable source of information. Verify his responses with family members, friends, or health care personnel. Also check hospital records from previous admissions, and compare his past behavior, symptoms, and circumstances with the current situation.

Explore the patient's chief complaint, current symptoms, psychiatric history, demographic data, socioeconomic data, cultural and religious beliefs, medication history, and physical illnesses, as follows.

Chief complaint

The patient may not voice his chief complaint directly. Instead, you or others may note that he is having difficulty coping or is exhibiting unusual behavior. If this occurs, determine whether the patient is aware of the problem. When documenting the patient's response, write it verbatim, and enclose it in quotation marks.

Current symptoms

Ask about the onset of symptoms, their severity and persistence, and whether they began abruptly. Compare the patient's condition with his normal level of functioning.

Psychiatric history

Discuss past psychiatric disturbances, such as episodes of delusions, violence, attempted suicides, drug or alcohol abuse, or depression, and previous psychiatric treatment.

Demographic data

Determine the patient's age, sex, ethnic origin, language, birthplace, religion, and marital status. Use this information to establish a baseline and validate the patient's record.

Socioeconomic data

Patients suffering hardships may show symptoms of distress during an illness. Information about your patient's educational level, housing conditions, income, employment status, and family may provide clues to his problem.

Cultural and religious beliefs

A patient's background and values affect his response to illness and his adaptation to care. Certain questions and behaviors considered inappropriate in one culture may be acceptable in another.

Medication history

Certain drugs can cause symptoms of mental illness. Review any medications the patient may be taking, including over-the-counter drugs, and check for interactions. If he's taking an antipsychotic, antidepressant, anxiolytic, or antimanic drug, ask if his symptoms have improved, if he's taking the medication as prescribed, and if he has had any adverse reactions.

Physical illnesses

Find out if the patient has a history of medical disorders that may cause disorientation, distorted thought processes, depression, or other symptoms of mental illness. Does he have a history of renal or hepatic failure, infection, thyroid disease, increased intracranial pressure, or a metabolic disorder?

Appearance, behavior, and mental status

Observe and record your appraisal of the patient's appearance, behavior, mood, thought processes, cognitive function, coping mechanisms, and potential for self-destructive behavior, as follows.

General
appearance

The patient's appearance helps to indicate his emotional and mental status. Specifically, note his dress and grooming. Is his appearance clean and appropriate to his age, sex, and situation? Is the patient's posture erect or slouched? Is his head lowered? What about his gait? Is it brisk, slow, shuffling, or unsteady? Does he walk normally? Note his facial expression. Does he look alert or does he stare blankly? Does he appear sad or angry? Does the patient maintain direct eye contact? Does he stare at you for long periods?

Behavior

Note the patient's demeanor and overall attitude as well as any extraordinary behavior such as speaking to a person who isn't present. Also record mannerisms. Does he bite his nails, fidget, or pace? Does he display any tics or tremors? How does he respond to the interviewer? Is he cooperative, friendly, hostile, or indifferent?

Mood

Does the patient appear excited or depressed? Is he crying, sweating, breathing heavily, or trembling? Ask him to describe his current feelings in concrete terms and to suggest possible reasons for these feelings. Note inconsistencies between body language and mood (such as smiling when discussing an anger-provoking situation).

Thought
processes and
cognitive
function

Evaluate the patient's orientation to time, place, and person. Look for delusions, hallucinations, obsessions, compulsions, fantasies, and daydreams. Check the patient's attention span and ability to recall events in both the distant and recent past. To assess immediate recall, ask him to repeat a series of five names of objects. Test his intellectual functioning by asking him to add a series of numbers; sensory perception and coordination, by having him copy a simple drawing. Inappropriate responses to a hypothetical situation ("What would you do if you won the lottery?") can indicate impaired judgment. Keep in mind that the patient's cultural background and personal values will influence his answer.

Note speech characteristics that may indicate altered thought processes, including monosyllabic responses, irrelevant or illogical replies to questions, convoluted or excessively detailed speech, repetitive speech, a flight of ideas, and sudden silence without an obvious reason.

Coping mechanisms defined

Coping, or defense, mechanisms help to relieve anxiety. Common ones include:
• **Denial.** Refusal to admit truth or reality.
• **Displacement.** Transference of an emotion from its original object to a substitute.
• **Fantasy.** Creation of unrealistic or improbable images to escape from daily pressures and responsibilities.
• **Identification.** Unconscious adoption of the personality characteristics, attitudes, values, and behavior of another person.

• **Projection.** Displacement of negative feelings onto another person.
• **Rationalization.** Substitution of acceptable reasons for the real or actual reasons motivating behavior.
• **Reaction formation.** Conduct in a manner opposite from the way the person feels.
• **Regression.** Return to behavior of an earlier, more comfortable time in life.
• **Repression.** Exclusion of unacceptable thoughts and feelings from the conscious mind, leaving them to operate in the subconscious.

Finally, evaluate the patient's degree of insight by asking if he understands the significance of his illness, the proposed treatment plan, and the effect it will have on his life.

Coping mechanisms

The patient who's faced with a stressful situation may adopt coping or defense mechanisms—behaviors that operate on an unconscious level to protect the ego. Examples include denial, regression, displacement, projection, reaction formation, and fantasy. (See *Coping mechanisms defined.*) Look for an excessive reliance on these coping mechanisms.

Potential for self-destructive behavior

Mentally healthy people may take death-defying risks, such as participating in dangerous sports. Risks taken by self-destructive patients aren't death-defying, but death-seeking.

Not all self-destructive behavior is suicidal in intent. Some patients engage in self-destructive behavior because it helps them feel alive. A patient who has lost touch with reality may cut or mutilate body parts to focus on physical pain, which may be less overwhelming than emotional distress.

Evaluate the patient for suicidal tendencies, particularly if he reports signs and symptoms of depression. (See *Suicide's warning signs.*) Not all such patients want to die; however, the incidence of suicide is higher in depressed patients than in patients with other diagnoses.

Suicide's warning signs

The following signs constitute suicidal behavior:
• withdrawal and social isolation
• signs and symptoms of depression, such as crying, fatigue, sadness, help-lessness, poor concentration, reduced interest in sex and other activities, con-stipation, and weight loss

• farewells to friends and family
• putting affairs in order
• giving away prized possessions
• covert suicide messages and death wishes
• obvious suicide messages such as "I'd be better off dead."

Diagnostic tests

The following tests provide information about mental status and physical causes of signs and symptoms.

Laboratory tests

Urinalysis, hemoglobin and hematocrit levels, serum electrolyte and serum glucose levels, and liver, kidney, and thyroid function tests screen for physical disorders that can cause psychiatric signs and symptoms. Toxicology studies of blood and urine can detect the presence of many drugs, and current laboratory methods can quantify the blood levels of these drugs. Patients on psychoactive drugs may need routine toxicology screening to ensure that they aren't receiving a toxic dose. (See *Toxicology screening,* page 10.)

Psychological and mental status tests

These tests evaluate the patient's mood, personality, and mental status. Frequently used tests include the following:
• The *Mini–Mental Status Examination* measures orientation, registration, recall, calculation, language, and graphomotor function.
• The *Cognitive Capacity Screening Examination* measures orientation, memory, calculation, and language.
• The *Cognitive Assessment Scale* measures orientation, general knowledge, mental ability, and psychomotor function.
• The *Global Deterioration Scale* assesses and stages primary degenerative dementia, based on orientation, memory, and neurologic function.
• The *Beck Depression Inventory* helps diagnose depression, determine its severity, and monitor response to treatment.
• The *Functional Dementia Scale* measures orientation, affect, and the ability to perform activities of daily living.
• The *Eating Attitudes Test* can reveal an eating disorder.

Toxicology screening

Toxic levels of certain drugs can be detected in blood, urine, or both.

Blood
• Alcohol (ethyl, isopropyl, and methyl)
• Ethchlorvynol (Placidyl)

Urine
• Chlorpromazine (Thorazine)
• Cocaine
• Desmethyldoxepin (metabolite of doxepin)
• Heroin (metabolized to and detected as morphine)
• Imipramine (Tofranil)
• Methadone
• Morphine
• Phencyclidine (PCP)

Blood and urine
• Acetaminophen
• Amitriptyline (Elavil)
• Amobarbital (Amytal)
• Butabarbital (Butisol)
• Butalbital (one component in Fiorinal)
• Caffeine
• Carisoprodol (Soma)

• Chlordiazepoxide (Librium)
• Codeine
• Desipramine (Pertofrane)
• Desmethyldiazepam (metabolite of diazepam)
• Diazepam (Valium)
• Diphenhydramine (Benadryl)
• Doxepin (Sinequan)
• Flurazepam (Dalmane)
• Glutethimide (Doriden)
• Ibuprofen (Medipren, Motrin)
• Meperidine (Demerol)
• Mephobarbital (Mebaral)
• Meprobamate (Equanil, Miltown)
• Methapyrilene
• Methaqualone (Quaalude)
• Methyprylon (Noludar)
• Norpropoxyphene (metabolite of propoxyphene)
• Nortriptyline (Aventyl)
• Oxazepam (Serax)
• Pentazocine (Talwin)
• Pentobarbital (Nembutal)
• Phenobarbital (Luminal)
• Propoxyphene (Darvon)
• Salicylates and their conjugates
• Secobarbital (Seconal)

• The *Minnesota Multiphasic Personality Inventory* helps assess personality traits and ego function in adolescents and adults. Test results include information on coping strategies, defenses, strengths, gender identification, and self-esteem. The test pattern may strongly suggest a diagnostic category, point to a suicide risk, or indicate the potential for violence.

EEG and brain imaging studies

Tests visualizing electrical brain-wave pattern disturbances or anatomic alterations screen for brain abnormalities.
• An *EEG* graphically records the brain's electrical activity. Abnormal results may indicate organic disease, psychotropic drug use, or certain psychological disorders.

• A *computed tomography (CT) scan* combines radiologic and computer analysis of tissue density to produce images of intracranial structures not readily seen on standard X-rays. This test can help detect brain contusions or calcifications, cerebral atrophy, hydrocephalus, inflammation, space-occupying lesions, and vascular abnormalities.

• A *magnetic resonance imaging (MRI) scan* is a noninvasive imaging technique. MRI localizes atomic nuclei that magnetically align and then fall out of alignment in response to a radio frequency pulse. The MRI scanner records signals from nuclei as they realign; it then translates the signals into detailed pictures of anatomic structures. Compared with conventional X-rays and CT scans, the MRI scan provides superior contrast of soft tissues and sharper differentiation of normal and abnormal tissues. It also provides images of multiple planes in regions where bones usually interface.

• A *positron emission tomography (PET) scan* provides colorimetric information about the brain's metabolic activity by detecting how quickly tissues consume radioactive isotopes. This test helps diagnose neuropsychiatric problems, such as Alzheimer's disease, and some mental illnesses.

Self-test questions

You can quickly review your comprehension of this introductory chapter by answering the following questions. The correct answers to these questions and their rationales appear on pages 153 and 154.

1. Which of the following factors have contributed to a rise in depression among elderly people?
   a. The struggle to cope with trauma
   b. The loss of effective support systems
   c. Faltering self-esteem
   d. Isolation, loneliness, and fear of violent crime

2. In the *DSM-IV* system of classifying mental disorders, which axis encompasses the patient's level of functioning?

    a. Axis II
    b. Axis III
    c. Axis IV
    d. Axis V

3. Socioeconomic data are important to a patient's history because:
    a. they establish a baseline.
    b. patients experiencing hardships are more likely to show distress.
    c. a patient's background and values affect his adaptation to care.
    d. they influence a patient's answers to questions.

4. Which of the following assessments provides clues to the patient's mood?
    a. Response to the interviewer
    b. Orientation to time, place, and person
    c. Description of his current feelings
    d. Questioning his understanding of the significance of his illness

5. Which of the following psychological and mental status tests measures orientation, general knowledge, mental ability, and psychomotor function?
    a. Cognitive Assessment Scale
    b. Cognitive Capacity Screening Examination
    c. Global Deterioration Scale
    d. Functional Dementia Scale

6. Which of the following studies may indicate psychotropic drug use?
    a. EEG
    b. CT scan
    c. MRI scan
    d. PET scan

CHAPTER 2

Disorders of Infancy, Childhood, and Adolescence

The disorders in this section typically become apparent before adulthood and can persist through it. They include mental retardation, which is transmitted genetically; tic disorders, which begin before age 21; autistic disorder, which usually becomes apparent before age 3; and attention-deficit hyperactivity disorder, which is difficult to diagnose before age 4 or 5.

Mental retardation

The American Association on Mental Retardation (AAMR) defines mental retardation as "significantly subaverage general intellectual function existing concurrently with deficits in adaptive behavior manifesting itself during the developmental period (before age 18)." An estimated 1% to 3% of the population is mentally retarded, demonstrating an IQ below 70 and an associated difficulty in carrying out tasks required for personal independence. Retardation commonly is accompanied by other physical and emotional disorders that may constitute handicaps in themselves. Mental retardation places a significant burden on patients and their families, resulting in stress, frustration, and family problems.

Causes of mental retardation

• Chromosomal abnormalities (Down's syndrome, Klinefelter's syndrome)
• Disorders resulting from unknown prenatal influences (hydrocephalus, hydranencephaly, microcephaly)
• Disorders of metabolism or nutrition (phenylketonuria, hypothyroidism, Hurler's syndrome, galactosemia, Tay-Sachs disease)
• Environmental influences (cultural-familial retardation, poor nutrition, lack of medical care)

• Gestational disorders (prematurity)
• Gross brain disorders that develop after birth (neurofibromatosis, intracranial neoplasm)
• Infection and intoxication (congenital rubella, syphilis, lead poisoning, meningitis, encephalitis, insecticides, drugs, maternal viral infection, toxins)
• Psychiatric disorders (autism)
• Trauma or physical agents (mechanical injury, asphyxia, hyperpyrexia)

Causes

A specific cause is identifiable in only 25% of mentally retarded people and, of these, only 10% have the potential for cure. In the remaining 75%, predisposing factors, such as deficient prenatal or perinatal care, inadequate nutrition, poor social environment, and poor child-rearing practices, contribute significantly to mental retardation. (See *Causes of mental retardation.*)

Prenatal screening for genetic defects (such as Tay-Sachs disease) and genetic counseling for families at risk for specific defects have reduced the incidence of genetically transmitted mental retardation.

Signs and symptoms

The observable effects of mental retardation are deviations from normal adaptive behaviors, ranging from learning disabilities and uncontrollable behavior to severe cognitive and motor skill impairment. The earlier a child's adaptive deficit is recognized and he's placed in a special learning program, the more likely he is to achieve age-appropriate adaptive behaviors. If the patient is older, review his adaptation to his environment.

The family of a patient who is mentally retarded may report many problems stemming from frustration, fear, and exhaustion. These problems, such as financial difficulties, abuse, and divorce, can compromise the child's care. Physical examination may reveal signs of abuse or neglect.

People who are mentally retarded may exhibit signs and symptoms of other disorders, such as cleft lip, cleft palate, congenital heart defects, and cerebral palsy, as well as a lowered resistance to infection.

Diagnosis

A score below 70 on a standardized IQ test confirms mental retardation. The recognized levels of mental retardation are as follows:
• mild retardation: IQ of 50–55 to approximately 70
• moderate retardation: IQ of 35–40 to 50–55
• severe retardation: IQ of 20–25 to 35–40
• profound retardation: IQ of less than 20–25.

The IQ test primarily predicts school performance and must be supplemented by other diagnostic evaluations.

For example, the Adaptive Behavior Scale deals with behaviors important to activities of daily living. This test evaluates self-help skills (toileting and eating), physical and social development, language, socialization, and time and number concepts. It also examines inappropriate behaviors (such as violent or destructive acts, withdrawal, and self-abusive or sexually aberrant behavior).

Age-appropriate adaptive behaviors are assessed by the use of developmental screening tests such as the Denver Developmental Screening test. These tests compare the subject's functional level with the normal level for the same chronological age. The greater the discrepancy between chronological and developmental age, the more severe the retardation.

In children, the functional level is based on sensorimotor skills, self-help skills, and socialization. In adolescents and adults, it is based on academic skills, reasoning and judgment skills, and social skills.

Treatment

Effective management requires an interdisciplinary team approach. A primary goal is to develop the patient's strengths as fully as possible. Another major goal is the development of social adaptive skills.

Mentally retarded children require special education and training, ideally beginning in infancy. An individualized, effective education program can optimize the quality of life for even the profoundly retarded.

The prognosis for people with mental retardation is related more to timing and aggressive treatment, personal motivation, training opportunities, and associated conditions than to the mental retardation itself. With good support systems, many mentally retarded people become productive members of society. Successful management leads to independent functioning and occupational skills for some and a sheltered environment for others.

Special considerations

• Support the parents of a child diagnosed with mental retardation. Not only may they be overwhelmed by caretaking and financial concerns, but they also may have difficulty accepting and bonding with their child.

• Remember that the child with mental retardation has all the ordinary needs of a normal child plus those created by his handicap. The child especially needs affection, acceptance, stimulation, and prudent, consistent discipline; he is less able to cope if rejected, overprotected, or forced beyond his abilities.

• When caring for a hospitalized retarded patient, promote continuity of care by acting as a liaison for parents and other health care professionals involved in his care.

• During hospitalization, continue training programs already in place, but remember that illness may bring on some regression.

• For the severely retarded child, suggest ways for parents to cope with the guilt, frustration, and exhaustion that often accompany caring for such a child. In particular, parents of a severely retarded child need an extensive teaching and discharge planning program, including physical care procedures, stress reduction techniques, support services, and referral to developmental programs. Request a social services consultation to investigate available community resources.

• Teach parents how to care for the special needs of the retarded child. Suggest that they contact the AAMR for information and referral.

• Teach retarded adolescents how to deal with the physical changes they are experiencing and sexual maturation. Encourage them to participate in appropriate sex education classes. A mentally retarded person may have difficulty expressing his sexual concerns because of limited verbal skills.

Tic disorders

Including Tourette syndrome, chronic motor or vocal tic disorder, and transient tic disorder, tic disorders are similar pathophysiologically but differ in severity and prognosis. All tic disorders, commonly known simply as "tics," are involuntary, spasmodic, recurrent, and purposeless motor movements or vocalizations.

These disorders are classified as motor or vocal and as simple or complex. According to the *DSM-IV*, motor and vocal tics are classified as simple or complex. However, category boundaries remain unclear. Also, combinations of tics may occur simultaneously.

Simple motor tics include eye blinking, neck jerking, shoulder shrugging, head banging, head turning, tongue protrusion, lip or tongue biting, nail biting, hair pulling, and facial grimacing. Some examples of complex motor tics are facial gestures, grooming behaviors, hitting or biting oneself, jumping, hopping, touching, squatting, deep knee bends, retracing steps, twirling when walking, stamping, smelling an object, and imitating the movements of someone who is being observed (echopraxia).

Examples of simple vocal tics include coughing, throat clearing, grunting, sniffing, snorting, hissing, clicking, yelping, and barking. Complex vocal tics may involve repeating words out of context; using socially unacceptable words, many of which are obscene (coprolalia); or repeating the last-heard sound, word, or phrase of another person (echolalia).

Tics begin before age 18. All tic disorders are three times more common in boys than in girls. Transient tics usually are self-limiting, but Tourette syndrome follows a chronic course with remissions and exacerbations.

Causes

Although their exact cause is unknown, tic disorders occur more frequently in certain families, suggesting a genetic cause. Tics commonly develop when a child experiences overwhelming anxiety, usually associated with normal maturation. Tics may be precipitated or exacerbated by the use of phenothiazines or central nervous system stimulants or by head trauma.

Signs and symptoms

Assessment findings vary according to the type of tic disorder. Inspection, coupled with the patient's history, may reveal the specific motor or vocal patterns that characterize the tic, as well as the frequency, complexity, and precipitating factors. The patient or his family may report that the tics occur sporadically many times a day.

Note whether certain situations exacerbate the tics. All tic disorders may be exacerbated by stress, and they usually diminish markedly during sleep. The patient also may report that they occur during activities that require concentration, such as reading or sewing.

Determine whether the patient can control the tics. Most patients can, with conscious effort, control them for short periods.

Psychosocial assessment may reveal underlying stressful factors, such as problems with social adjustment, lack of self-esteem, and depression.

Diagnosis

For characteristic findings in patients with this condition, see *Diagnosing tic disorders.*

Treatment

Behavior modification techniques and operant conditioning help treat some tic disorders. Psychotherapy can help the patient uncover underlying conflicts and issues as well as deal with the problems caused by the tics. Tourette syndrome is best treated with medications and psychotherapy.

No medications are helpful in treating transient tics. Haloperidol is the drug of choice for Tourette syndrome. Pimozide (an oral dopamine-blocking drug) and clonidine are alternative choices. Antianxiety agents may be useful in dealing with secondary anxiety but do not reduce the severity or frequency of the tics. (For information about related stress disorders, see *Stress disorders with physical manifestations,* page 20.)

Special considerations

• Offer emotional support and help the patient prevent fatigue.
• Suggest that the patient with Tourette syndrome contact the Tourette Syndrome Association for information and support.

Diagnosing tic disorders

The diagnosis of a tic disorder is based on fulfillment of the criteria documented in the *DSM-IV.*

Tourette syndrome
• The person has had multiple motor tics and one or more vocal tics at some time during the illness, although not necessarily concurrently.
• The tics occur many times a day (usually in bouts) nearly every day or intermittently for more than 1 year.
• The disturbance causes marked distress or significant impairment in social, occupational, or other important areas of functioning.
• Onset occurs before age 18.
• The disturbance is not the direct physiologic effect of a substance or a general medical condition.

Chronic motor or vocal tic disorder
• The person has had single or multiple motor or vocal tics, but not both, at some time during the illness.
• The tics occur many times a day nearly every day or intermittently for more than 1 year, and during this period the person has never had a tic-free period exceeding 3 consecutive months.

• The disturbance causes marked distress or significant impairment in social, occupational, or other important areas of functioning.
• Onset occurs before age 18.
• The disturbance is not the direct physiologic effect of a substance or a general medical condition.
• Criteria have never been met for Tourette syndrome.

Transient tic disorder
• The person has single or multiple motor or vocal tics, or both.
• The tics occur many times a day nearly every day for at least 4 weeks, but for no longer than 12 consecutive months.
• The disturbance causes marked distress or significant impairment in social, occupational, or other important areas of functioning.
• Onset occurs before age 18.
• The disturbance is not the direct physiologic effect of a substance or a general medical condition.
• Criteria have never been met for Tourette syndrome or chronic motor or vocal tic disorder.

• Help the patient identify and eliminate any avoidable stress and learn positive new ways to deal with anxiety.
• Encourage the patient to verbalize his feelings about his illness. Help him understand that the movements are involuntary and that he shouldn't feel guilty or blame himself.

Stress disorders with physical manifestations

In addition to tic disorders, other stress-related disorders that produce physical signs in children include stuttering, functional enuresis, functional encopresis, sleepwalking, and sleep terrors.

Stuttering

This disorder, characterized by abnormalities of speech rhythms with repetitions and hesitations at the beginning of words, also may involve movements of the respiratory muscles, shoulders, and face.

Stuttering may be associated with mental dullness, poor social background, and a history of birth trauma. This disorder most commonly occurs in children of average or superior intelligence who fear they can't meet the expectations of their families.

Related problems may include low self-esteem, tension, anxiety, humiliation, and withdrawal from social situations.

About 80% of stutterers recover after age 16. Evaluation and treatment by a speech pathologist teaches the stutterer to place equal weight on each syllable in a sentence, how to breathe properly, and how to control anxiety.

Functional enuresis

This disorder is characterized by intentional or involuntary voiding of urine, usually during the night (nocturnal enuresis).

Considered normal in children until age 3 or 4, functional enuresis occurs in about 40% of children at this age and persists in 10% to age 5, in 5% to age 10, and in 1% of boys to age 18. The disorder persists longer in boys.

Causes may be related to stress in the child's life, such as the birth of a sibling, the move to a new home, divorce, separation, hospitalization, faulty toilet training (inconsistent, demanding, or punitive), and unrealistic responsibilities.

Associated problems include low self-esteem, social withdrawal from peers because of ostracism and ridicule, and anger, rejection, and punishment by caregivers.

Advise parents to avoid punishing the child. A matter-of-fact attitude helps the child learn to control his bladder function without undue stress.

If enuresis persists into late childhood, treatment with imipramine may help. Dry-bed therapy may include the use of an alarm apparatus (wet bell pad), social motivation, self-correction of accidents, and positive reinforcement.

Functional encopresis

Denoted by evacuation of feces into the child's clothes or inappropriate receptacles, functional encopresis is associated with low intelligence, cerebral dysfunction, or other developmental symptoms such as language lag. Some children also show inefficient and ineffective gastric motility.

Related problems may include repressed anger, withdrawal from peers in social relationships, and loss of self-esteem.

Treatment involves encouraging the child to come to his parents when he has an "accident." Encourage parents to help the child by giving him clean clothes without criticism or punishment. Medical examination should rule out any physical disorder. Child, adult, and family therapy may help reduce anger and disappointment in the child's development and improve parenting techniques.

Stress disorders with physical manifestations *(continued)*

Sleepwalking and sleep terrors
In sleepwalking, the child calmly rises from bed in a state of altered consciousness and walks about with no subsequent recollection of any dream content. In sleep terrors, he awakes terrified, in a state of clouded consciousness, often unable to recognize parents and familiar surroundings. Visual hallucinations are common.

Sleepwalking is usually a response to an emotional concern.

Sleep terrors are a normal developmental event in 2- and 3-year-old children, usually occurring within 30 minutes to 3½ hours of sleep onset. Tachycardia, tachypnea, diaphoresis, dilated pupils, and piloerection are associated with sleep terrors. The child also may fear being alone.

Tell parents to make sure the child has access to them at night. Sleep terrors usually are self-limiting and subside within a few weeks.

Parents should be told to gently "talk" the sleepwalking child back to his bed. If the child wakes, they should be comforting and supportive, not teasing.

Autistic disorder

A severe, pervasive developmental disorder, autistic disorder is marked by unresponsiveness to social contact, gross deficits in intelligence and language development, ritualistic and compulsive behaviors, restricted capacity for developmentally appropriate activities and interests, and bizarre responses to the environment. (For more information about similar disorders in this class, see *Other pervasive developmental disorders,* page 22.) Autistic disorder may be complicated by epileptic seizures, depression and, during periods of stress, catatonic phenomena. Autism usually becomes apparent before the child reaches age 30 months but, in some children, the actual onset is difficult to determine. Occasionally, autistic disorder isn't recognized until the child enters school. Autistic disorder is rare, affecting 4 to 5 children per 10,000 births. It affects three to four times more boys than girls, usually the firstborn boy. The prognosis is poor; most patients require a structured environment throughout life.

Causes

The causes of autistic disorder remain unclear but are thought to include psychological, physiologic, and sociological factors. The parents of an autistic child may appear dis-

Other pervasive developmental disorders

Although autistic disorder is the most severe and most typical of the pervasive developmental disorders, recent evidence points to other, similar disorders in this class.

For example, the *DSM-IV's* category *pervasive developmental disorder not otherwise specified* refers to those patients who don't meet the criteria for autistic disorder but who *do* exhibit impaired development of reciprocal social interaction and of verbal and nonverbal communication skills.

Some patients with this diagnosis exhibit a markedly restricted repertoire of activities and interests, but others don't. Research suggests that these disorders are more common than autistic disorder, occurring in 6 to 10 of every 10,000 children.

tant and unaffectionate. However, because autistic children are unresponsive or respond with rigid, screaming resistance to touch and attention, parental remoteness may be merely a frustrated, helpless reaction to this disorder, not its cause.

Some autistic children show abnormal but nonspecific EEG findings that suggest brain dysfunction, possibly resulting from trauma, disease, or structural abnormality. Autistic disorder also has been associated with maternal rubella, untreated phenylketonuria, tuberous sclerosis, anoxia during birth, encephalitis, infantile spasms, and fragile X syndrome.

Signs and symptoms

A primary characteristic of infantile autistic disorder is unresponsiveness to people. Infants with this disorder won't cuddle, avoid eye contact and facial expression, and are indifferent to affection and physical contact. Parents may report that the child becomes rigid or flaccid when held, cries when touched, and shows little or no interest in human contact.

As the infant grows older, his smiling response is delayed or absent. He doesn't lift his arms in anticipation of being picked up or form an attachment to a specific caregiver. Nor does he show the anxiety about strangers that's typical in the 8-month-old infant.

The autistic child fails to learn the usual socialization games (peek-a-boo, pat-a-cake, or bye-bye). He's likely to relate to others only to fill a physical need and then without eye contact or speech. The end result may be mutual withdrawal between parents and child.

Severe language impairment and lack of imaginative play are characteristic. The child may be mute or may use immature speech patterns. For example, he may use a single word to express a series of activities; he may say "ground" when referring to any step in using a playground slide.

His speech commonly shows echolalia (meaningless repetition of words or phrases addressed to him) and pronoun reversal ("you go walk" when he means "I want to go for a walk"). When answering a question, he may simply repeat the question to mean yes and remain silent to mean no.

He shows little imagination, seldom acting out adult roles or engaging in fantasy play. In fact, he may insist on lining up an exact number of toys in the same manner over and over or repetitively mimic the actions of someone else.

The autistic child shows characteristically bizarre behavior patterns, such as screaming fits, rituals, rhythmic rocking, arm flapping, crying without tears, and disturbed sleeping and eating patterns. His behavior may be self-destructive (hand biting, eye gouging, hair pulling, or head banging) or self-stimulating (playing with his own saliva, feces, and urine).

His bizarre responses to his environment include an extreme compulsion for sameness.

In response to sensory stimuli, the autistic child may underreact or overreact; he may ignore objects—dropping those he is given or not looking at them—or he may become excessively absorbed in them—continually watching the objects or the movement of his own fingers over the objects. He commonly responds to stimuli by head banging, rocking, whirling, and hand flapping. He tends to avoid using sight and hearing to interact with the environment.

The autistic child may exhibit additional behavioral abnormalities, such as:
• cognitive impairment (most have an IQ of 35 to 49)
• eating, drinking, and sleeping problems—for example, limiting his diet to just a few foods, excessive drinking, or repeatedly waking during the night and rocking
• mood disorders, including labile mood, giggling or crying without reason, lack of emotional responses, no fear of real danger but excessive fear of harmless objects, and generalized anxiety.

Diagnosing autistic disorder

A diagnosis of autistic disorder is made when the patient meets the criteria set forth in the *DSM-IV.* At least six of the following characteristics from the social interaction, communication, and patterns categories must be present, including at least two characteristics from the social interaction category and one each from the communication and patterns categories:

Social interaction
Qualitative impairment in social interaction as manifested by at least two of the following:
• marked impairment in the use of multiple nonverbal behaviors, such as eye-to-eye gaze, facial expression, body postures, and gestures to regulate social interaction
• failure to develop peer relationships appropriate to developmental level
• lack of spontaneous seeking to share enjoyment, interests, or achievements with other people
• lack of social or emotional reciprocity
• gross impairment in ability to make peer friendships.

Communication
Qualitative impairment in communication, as manifested by at least one of the following:
• delay in, or total lack of, spoken language development
• in individuals with adequate speech, marked impairment in initiating or sustaining a conversation with others
• stereotyped and repetitive use of language or idiosyncratic language
• lack of varied, spontaneous make-believe play or social imitative play appropriate to developmental level.

Patterns
Restricted, repetitive, and stereotyped patterns of behavior, interests, and activities, as manifested by at least one of the following:
• encompassing preoccupation with one or more stereotyped and restricted patterns of interest that is abnormal either in intensity or focus
• apparently inflexible adherence to specific nonfunctional routines or rituals
• stereotyped and repetitive motor mannerisms
• persistent preoccupation with parts of objects.

Additional criteria
Delays or abnormal functioning in at least one of the following areas, with onset before age 3:
• social interaction
• language as used in social communication
• symbolic or imaginative play
    The disturbance is not better accounted for by Rett's syndrome or childhood disintegrative disorder.

Diagnosis

For characteristic findings in patients with this condition, see *Diagnosing autistic disorder.*

Treatment

The difficult and prolonged treatment of autistic disorder must begin early, continue for years (through adolescence), and coordinate efforts to encourage social adjustment and speech development and to reduce self-destructive behavior.

Behavioral techniques are used to decrease symptoms and increase the child's ability to respond. Positive reinforcement, using food and other rewards, can enhance language and social skills. Providing pleasurable sensory and motor stimulation (jogging, playing with a ball) encourages appropriate behavior and helps eliminate inappropriate behavior. Pharmacologic intervention with an agent such as haloperidol may be helpful.

Treatment may take place in a psychiatric institution, in a specialized school, or in a day-care program, but the current trend is toward home treatment. Because family members tend to feel inadequate and guilty, they may need counseling. Until the causes of infantile autism are known, prevention is not possible.

Special considerations

• Reduce self-destructive behaviors. Physically stop the child from harming himself, while firmly saying "no." When he responds to your voice, first give a primary reward (such as food); later, substitute verbal or physical reinforcement (such as "good," or a hug or a pat on the back).
• Foster appropriate use of language. Provide positive reinforcement when the child indicates his needs correctly. Give verbal reinforcement at first (such as "good" or "great"); later, give physical reinforcement (such as a hug or a pat on the hand or shoulder).
• Encourage development of self-esteem. Show the child that he's acceptable as a person.
• Encourage self-care. For example, place a brush in the child's hand and guide his hand to brush his hair. Similarly, teach him to wash his hands and face.
• Encourage acceptance of minor environmental changes. Prepare the child for the change by telling him about it. Make the change minor—for example, change the color of his bedspread or the placement of food on his plate. When he has accepted minor changes, move on to bigger ones.
• Provide emotional support to the parents, and refer them to the Autism Society of America.
• Teach the parents how to physically care for the child's needs.
• Teach the parents how to identify signs of excessive stress and coping skills to use under these circumstances. Emphasize that they'll be ineffective caregivers if they don't take the time to meet their own needs in addition to those of their child.

> • Help the parents understand that they aren't responsible for the child's condition.

Attention-deficit hyperactivity disorder

This disorder is characterized by difficulty in focusing attention or engaging in quiet, passive activities, or both. Although the disorder is present at birth, diagnosis before age 5 is difficult unless the child shows severe symptoms. (Some patients, in fact, aren't diagnosed until adulthood). Males are three times more likely to be affected than females.

Causes

Attention-deficit hyperactivity disorder is commonly thought to be a physiologic brain disorder, with a tendency to occur in families. Some studies indicate the disorder may be caused by disturbances in neurotransmitter levels.

Signs and symptoms

Typically, the patient with attention-deficit disorder is characterized as a fidgeter and a daydreamer. He may also be considered inattentive, lazy, or incapable of hard work. Although the patient may be intelligent, his school or work performance patterns are sporadic, and he may jump from one project, thought, or task to another without completing anything.

Some patients have an attention deficit without hyperactivity. They're less likely to be diagnosed and treated.

In a younger child, signs and symptoms include an inability to wait in line, remain seated, wait his turn, or concentrate on one activity until its completion. In an older child or adult, they include impulsiveness, inability to avoid distractions, emotional lability, inattentiveness, or daydreaming. Pervasive disorganization causes difficulty meeting deadlines and keeping track of school or work materials.

Diagnosis

Commonly, the child with attention-deficit hyperactivity disorder is referred for evaluation by the school—with the problems reflecting the child's age. Diagnosis of this disorder usually begins by obtaining data from several sources. Parents, teachers, and the person are interviewed. Complete psychological, medical, and neurologic evaluations are performed to rule out other problems. Then the child takes tests that measure impulsiveness, attention, and ability to sustain a task. The combined findings portray a picture of the disorder and of the areas of support he'll need.

For characteristic findings in patients with this condition, see *Diagnosing attention-deficit hyperactivity disorder*, page 28.

Treatment

Education is the first step. Everyone on the treatment team (which ideally includes parents, teachers, and therapists as well as the patient and the doctor) must understand the disorder and its effect on the patient's functioning.

Treatment varies depending on the severity of symptoms and their impact on the patient's ability to function. Behavior modification, coaching, external structure, use of planning and organizing systems, and supportive psychotherapy help the patient cope with the disorder.

Some patients benefit from medication to decrease symptoms. Ideally, the treatment team identifies the symptoms to be managed, selects medication, and then tracks the patient's symptoms to determine the effectiveness of the medication. Stimulants, such as methylphenidate and dexedrine, are commonly used. Other agents, including tricyclic antidepressants (such as desipramine and nortriptyline), mood stabilizers, and beta blockers may also help control symptoms.

Special considerations

• Help the patient develop external structure and controls.
• Set realistic expectations and limits because the patient is easily frustrated (which leads to decreased self-control).
• Remain calm and consistent. Keep instructions short and simple.
• Provide praise, rewards, and positive feedback.

Diagnosing attention-deficit hyperactivity disorder

The *DSM-IV* groups a selection of symptoms into inattention and hyperactivity-impulsivity categories. The diagnosis of attention-deficit hyperactivity disorder is based on the person demonstrating at least six symptoms from the inattention group or at least six symptoms from the hyperactivity-impulsivity group. The symptoms must have persisted for at least 6 months to a degree that is maladaptive and inconsistent with developmental level.

Symptoms of inattention
The person manifesting *inattention:*
• often fails to give close attention to details or makes careless mistakes in schoolwork, work, or other activities
• often has difficulty sustaining attention in tasks or play activities
• often does not seem to listen when spoken to directly
• often does not follow through on instructions and fails to finish schoolwork, chores, or duties in the workplace (not because of oppositional behavior or failure to understand instructions)
• often has difficulty organizing tasks and activities
• often avoids, dislikes, or is reluctant to engage in tasks that require sustained mental effort (such as schoolwork or homework)
• often loses things necessary for tasks or activities (for example, toys, school assignments, pencils, books, or tools)
• often becomes distracted by extraneous stimuli
• often demonstrates forgetfulness in daily activities.

Symptoms of hyperactivity-impulsivity
The person manifesting *hyperactivity:*
• often fidgets with hands or feet or squirms in seat
• often leaves seat in classroom or in other situations in which remaining seated is expected
• often runs about or climbs excessively in situations in which remaining seated is expected
• often has difficulty playing or engaging in leisure activities quietly
• often characterized as "on the go" or often acts as if "driven by a motor"
• often talks excessively.
   The person manifesting *impulsivity:*
• often blurts out answers before questions have been completed
• often has difficulty awaiting his turn
• often interrupts or intrudes on others.

Additional features
• Some hyperactivity-impulsivity or inattention symptoms that cause impairment are evident before age 7.
• Some impairment from symptoms is present in two or more settings.
• Clinically significant impairment in social, academic, or occupational functioning must be clearly evident.
• The symptoms do not occur exclusively during the course of a pervasive developmental disorder, schizophrenia, or other psychotic disorder and are not better accounted for by another mental disorder.

Self-test questions

You can review your comprehension of this chapter on the disorders of infancy, childhood, and adolescence by answering the following questions. The answers to these questions and their rationales appear on pages 154 to 156.

1. The recognized IQ level for moderate mental retardation is:
   a. 50–55 to approximately 70.
   b. 35–40 to 50–55.
   c. 20–25 to 35–40.
   d. less than 20–25.

2. A primary goal of mental retardation treatment is:
   a. special education and training.
   b. promoting continuity of care.
   c. assisting parents to cope with concerns about their child's care.
   d. to fully develop the patient's strengths.

Case history
questions

Jim Boyle, age 19, has been diagnosed with Tourette syndrome.

3. One of the differential diagnostic criteria is that:
   a. tics occur many times a day nearly every day for at least 4 weeks, but no longer than 1 year.
   b. single or multiple motor or vocal tics, but not both, have been present at some time during the illness.
   c. tics occur many times a day (usually in bouts) nearly every day or intermittently for over a year.
   d. the disturbance causes marked distress or significant impairment in social, occupational, or other important areas of functioning.

4. Jim is most likely to be treated with:
   a. antianxiety agents.
   b. clonidine.
   c. pimozide.
   d. haloperidol.

Anthony Parker, age 3, has been diagnosed with autistic disorder.

5. Anthony exhibits marked impairment in the use of multiple nonverbal behaviors, a characteristic of:
   a. qualitative impairment in social interaction.
   b. qualitative impairment in communication.
   c. restrictive, repetitive, and stereotyped behavior patterns.
   d. abnormal functioning in language as used in social communication.

6. Reducing Anthony's self-destructive behavior is best accomplished by:
   a. distracting him and providing a food reward.
   b. substituting pleasurable sensory or motor stimulation.
   c. physically stopping the harmful action, while saying "no."
   d. distracting him and rewarding him with a hug.

Brian Languille, age 4, has been referred by his pre-kindergarten teacher and school guidance counselor for evaluation for attention-deficit hyperactivity disorder.

7. Which of the following would Brian's teacher cite?
   a. Brian hands in work late.
   b. He never knows where his crayons are.
   c. He's disorganized.
   d. He can't seem to wait in line or stay seated.

8. The treatment team feels Brian may benefit from drug therapy. To determine its effectiveness you should:
   a. evaluate inattention criteria.
   b. evaluate hyperactivity criteria.
   c. evaluate impulsivity criteria.
   d. identify and track particular symptoms.

CHAPTER 3

Psychoactive Substance Abuse

This section includes disorders, such as alcoholism and psychoactive drug abuse and dependence, that affect the central nervous system and cause physical and mental harm.

Alcoholism

A chronic disorder, alcoholism most often is described as uncontrolled intake of alcoholic beverages that interferes with physical and mental health, social and familial relationships, and occupational responsibilities. Alcoholism cuts across all social and economic groups, involves both sexes, and occurs at all stages of the life cycle, beginning as early as elementary school age. About 13% of all adults over age 18 have suffered from alcohol abuse or dependence at some time in their lives. The prevalence of drinking is highest between the ages of 21 and 34, but current statistics show that up to 19% of 12-year-olds to 17-year-olds have a serious drinking problem. Males are two to five times more likely to abuse alcohol than are females. According to some statistics, alcohol abuse is a factor in 60% of all automobile accidents.

Causes

Numerous biological, psychological, and sociocultural factors appear to be involved in alcohol addiction. An offspring of one alcoholic parent is seven to eight times more likely to become an alcoholic than is a peer without such a parent. Biological factors may include genetic or biochemical abnormalities, nutritional deficiencies, endocrine imbalances, and allergic responses.

Psychological factors may include the urge to drink alcohol to reduce anxiety or symptoms of mental illness; the desire to avoid responsibility in familial, social, and work relationships; and the need to bolster self-esteem.

Sociocultural factors include the availability of alcoholic beverages, group or peer pressure, an excessively stressful lifestyle, and social attitudes that approve of frequent drinking.

Signs and symptoms

Because people with alcohol dependence may hide or deny their addiction and may temporarily manage to maintain a functional life, assessing for alcoholism can be difficult. Note physical and psychosocial symptoms that suggest alcoholism. For example, the patient's history may suggest a need for daily or episodic alcohol use to maintain adequate functioning, an inability to discontinue or reduce alcohol intake, episodes of anesthesia or amnesia during intoxication (blackouts), episodes of violence during intoxication, and interference with social and familial relationships and occupational responsibilities.

Many minor complaints may be alcohol-related. The patient may report malaise, dyspepsia, mood swings or depression, and an increased incidence of infection. Observe the patient for poor personal hygiene and untreated injuries, such as cigarette burns, fractures, and bruises, that he can't fully explain. Note any evidence of an unusually high tolerance for sedatives and narcotics.

Watch for secretive behavior. Suspect alcoholism if the patient uses inordinate amounts of after-shave lotion or mouthwash.

When confronted, the patient may deny or rationalize the problem. Alternatively, he may be guarded or hostile in his response and may even sign out of the hospital against medical advice. He also may project his anger or feelings of guilt or inadequacy onto others to avoid confronting his illness.

Chronic alcohol abuse brings with it an array of physical complications. Assess for these complications in a patient with an alcohol-related disorder. (See *Complications of alcohol use.*)

Complications of alcohol use

Alcohol can damage body tissues by its direct irritating effects, by changes that take place in the body during its metabolism, by aggravation of existing disease, by accidents occurring during intoxication, and by interactions between the substance and drugs. Such tissue damage can cause the following complications.

Cardiopulmonary complications
• Cardiac arrhythmias
• Cardiomyopathy
• Chronic obstructive pulmonary disease
• Essential hypertension
• Increased risk of tuberculosis
• Pneumonia

Hepatic complications
• Alcoholic hepatitis
• Cirrhosis
• Fatty liver

GI complications
• Chronic diarrhea
• Esophageal cancer
• Esophageal varices
• Esophagitis
• Gastric ulcers

• Gastritis
• GI bleeding
• Malabsorption
• Pancreatitis

Neurologic complications
• Alcoholic dementia
• Alcoholic hallucinosis
• Alcohol withdrawal delirium
• Korsakoff's syndrome
• Peripheral neuropathy
• Seizure disorders
• Subdural hematoma
• Wernicke's encephalopathy

Psychiatric complications
• Amotivational syndrome
• Depression
• Fetal alcohol syndrome
• Impaired social and occupational functioning
• Multiple substance abuse
• Suicide

Other complications
• Beriberi
• Hypoglycemia
• Leg and foot ulcers
• Prostatitis

After abstinence or reduction of alcohol intake, manifestations of withdrawal—which begin shortly after drinking has stopped and last for 5 to 7 days—may vary. (See *Signs and symptoms of alcohol withdrawal*, page 34.)

The patient initially experiences anorexia, nausea, anxiety, fever, insomnia, diaphoresis, and tremors, progressing to severe tremulousness, agitation and, possibly, hallucinations and violent behavior. Major motor seizures can occur during withdrawal. Suspect alcoholism in unexplained seizure activity. For findings in alcoholism, see *Diagnosing substance dependence and related disorders*, pages 35 and 36.

(*Text continues on page 36.*)

Signs and symptoms of alcohol withdrawal

Withdrawal signs and symptoms may vary in degree from mild (morning hangover) to severe (alcohol withdrawal delirium). Formerly known as delirium tremens (DTs), alcohol withdrawal delirium is marked by acute distress following abrupt withdrawal after prolonged or massive use.

SIGNS AND SYMPTOMS	MILD	MODERATE	SEVERE
Motor impairment	Hand tremor	Visible tremors	Gross, uncontrollable bodily shaking
Anxiety	Mild restlessness	Obvious motor restlessness and anxiety	Extreme restlessness and agitation with intense fearfulness
Sleep disturbance	Restless sleep or insomnia	Marked insomnia and nightmares	Total wakefulness
Appetite	Impaired appetite	Marked anorexia	Rejection of all food and fluid except alcohol
GI symptoms	Nausea	Nausea and vomiting	Dry heaves and vomiting
Confusion	None	Variable	Marked confusion and disorientation
Hallucinations	None	Vague, transient visual and auditory hallucinations and illusions; commonly nocturnal	Visual and occasional auditory hallucinations, usually of fearful or threatening content; misidentification of people and frightening delusions related to hallucinatory experiences
Pulse rate	Tachycardia	Pulse rate of 100 to 120 beats/minute	Pulse rate of 120 to 140 beats/minute
Blood pressure	Normal or slightly elevated systolic	Usually elevated systolic	Elevated systolic and diastolic
Sweating	Slight	Obvious	Marked hyperhidrosis
Seizures	None	Possible	Common

Diagnosing substance dependence and related disorders

The *DSM-IV* identifies the diagnostic criteria for substance dependence, abuse, intoxication, and withdrawal as follows.

Substance dependence

• A maladaptive pattern of substance use leading to clinically significant impairment or distress, as manifested by three or more of the following criteria, occurring at any time within the same 12-month period:
— Tolerance, as defined by either of the following: the need for increased amounts of the substance to achieve intoxication or desired effect or a markedly diminished effect with continued use of the same amount of the substance
— Withdrawal, as manifested by either of the following: the characteristic withdrawal syndrome for the substance or use of the same, or similar, substance to relieve or avoid withdrawal symptoms
— The person often takes the substance in larger amounts or over a longer period than was intended.
— The person experiences a persistent desire or unsuccessful efforts to cut down or control substance use.
— The person spends a great deal of time in activities needed to obtain the substance, use the substance, or recover from its effects.
— The person abandons or reduces important social, occupational, or recreational activities because of substance use.
— The person continues using the substance despite knowledge of having a persistent or recurrent physical or psychological problem that is likely to have

been caused or exacerbated by the substance.

Substance abuse

• A maladaptive pattern of substance use leading to clinically significant impairment or distress, as manifested by one or more of the following, occurring within a 12-month period:
— Recurrent substance use resulting in a failure to fulfill major role obligations at work, school, or home
— Recurrent substance use in situations in which using the substance is physically hazardous
— Recurrent substance-related legal problems
— Continued substance use despite having persistent or recurrent social or interpersonal problems caused or exacerbated by the effects of the substance.
• Symptoms have never met the criteria for substance dependence for this class of substance.

Substance intoxication

• Development of a reversible substance-specific syndrome resulting from recent ingestion of, or exposure to, a substance
• Clinically significant maladaptive behavioral or psychological changes resulting from the effect of the substance on the central nervous system and developing during or shortly after use of the substance
• Symptoms not caused by a general medical condition and not better accounted for by another mental disorder.

(continued)

Diagnosing substance dependence and related disorders *(continued)*

Substance withdrawal
• Development of a substance-specific syndrome resulting from the cessation or reduction of substance use that has been heavy and prolonged
• Substance-specific syndrome causing clinically significant distress or impair-

ment in social, occupational, or other important areas of functioning
• Symptoms not caused by a general medical condition and not better accounted for by another mental disorder.

Diagnosis

Besides the diagnostic criteria posed in the *Diagnostic and Statistical Manual of Mental Disorders,* 4th edition *(DSM-IV),* clinical findings may support the diagnosis of alcoholism. Laboratory tests can confirm alcohol use and complications. For example, laboratory data can document recent alcohol ingestion. A blood alcohol level of 0.10% weight/volume (200 mg/dl) is accepted as the level of intoxication. Serum electrolyte studies may identify characteristic electrolyte abnormalities (in severe hepatic disease, the blood urea nitrogen level is increased and the serum glucose level is decreased).

Further testing may reveal increased serum ammonia and serum amylase levels. Urine toxicology may help to determine if the patient with alcohol withdrawal delirium or another acute complication abuses other drugs as well.

Liver function studies revealing increased levels of serum cholesterol, lactate dehydrogenase, alanine aminotransferase, aspartate aminotransferase, and creatine kinase may point to liver damage, and elevated serum amylase and lipase levels point to acute pancreatitis. A hematologic workup can identify anemia, thrombocytopenia, increased prothrombin time, and increased partial thromboplastin time.

Treatment

Total abstinence from alcohol is the only effective treatment. Supportive programs that offer detoxification, rehabilitation, and aftercare, including continued involvement in Alcoholics Anonymous (AA), may produce good long-term results.

Acute intoxication is treated symptomatically by supporting respiration, preventing aspiration of vomitus, replacing fluids, administering I.V. glucose to prevent hypoglycemia, correcting hypothermia or acidosis, and initiating emergency treatment for trauma, infection, or GI bleeding.

Treatment of chronic alcoholism relies on medications to deter alcohol use and treat effects of withdrawal; psychotherapy, consisting of behavior modification techniques, group therapy, and family therapy; and appropriate measures to relieve associated physical problems.

Aversion, or deterrent, therapy involves a daily oral dose of disulfiram to prevent compulsive drinking. This drug interferes with alcohol metabolism and allows toxic levels of acetaldehyde to accumulate in the patient's blood, producing immediate and potentially fatal distress if the patient consumes alcohol up to 2 weeks after taking it. Disulfiram is contraindicated during pregnancy and in patients with diabetes, heart disease, severe hepatic disease, or any disorder in which such a reaction could be especially dangerous. Another form of aversion therapy attempts to induce aversion by administering alcohol with an emetic.

For long-term success, the recovering individual must learn to fill the place alcohol once occupied in his life with something constructive. Aversion therapy with disulfiram may only substitute one drug dependence for another, so it should be used prudently.

Tranquilizers, particularly the benzodiazepines, occasionally are used to relieve overwhelming anxiety during rehabilitation. However, these drugs have addictive potential (substituting one substance abuse problem for another), and they can precipitate coma or even death when combined with alcohol. Phenothiazines and other antipsychotics are prescribed to control hyperactivity and psychosis. Anticonvulsants, antiemetics, and antidiarrheals also are used to treat symptoms of alcohol withdrawal.

Supportive counseling or individual, group, or family psychotherapy may help. Ongoing support groups are also helpful. In AA, a self-help group with more than a million members worldwide, the alcoholic finds emotional support from others with similar problems. About 40% of AA's members stay sober as long as 5 years, and 30% stay sober longer than that.

Special considerations

• During acute intoxication or withdrawal, carefully monitor the patient's mental status, heart rate, breath sounds, blood pressure, and temperature every 30 minutes to 6 hours.

• Evaluate the patient for signs of inadequate nutrition and dehydration. Institute seizure precautions and administer drugs prescribed to treat the signs and symptoms of withdrawal in chronic alcohol abuse.

• During withdrawal, orient the patient to reality because he may have hallucinations and may try to harm himself or others. Maintain a calm environment, minimizing noise and shadows to reduce the incidence of delusions and hallucinations. Avoid restraining the patient unless necessary to protect him or others.

• Approach the patient in a nonthreatening way. Limit sustained eye contact. Even if he's verbally abusive, listen attentively and respond with empathy. Explain all procedures.

• Monitor the patient for signs of depression or impending suicide.

• In chronic alcoholism, help the patient accept his drinking problem and the necessity for abstinence. Confront him about his behavior, urging him to examine his actions more realistically.

• If the patient is taking disulfiram (or has taken it within the past 2 weeks), warn him of the effects of alcohol ingestion, which may last from 30 minutes to 3 hours or longer. The reaction includes nausea, vomiting, facial flushing, headache, shortness of breath, red eyes, blurred vision, sweating, tachycardia, hypotension, and fainting. Emphasize that even a small amount of alcohol will induce this adverse reaction and that the longer he takes the drug, the greater his sensitivity to alcohol will be. Because of this, he must avoid even medicinal sources of alcohol, such as mouthwash, cough syrups, liquid vitamins, and cold remedies.

• Refer the patient to AA and offer to arrange a visit from an AA member. Stress the effectiveness of this organization.

• For individuals who have lost all contact with family and friends and who have a long history of unemployment, trouble with the law, or other problems associated with alcohol abuse, rehabilitation may involve job training, sheltered workshops, halfway houses, and other supervised facilities.

• Refer spouses of alcoholics to Al-Anon and children of alcholics to Alateen. By participating in these self-help groups,

family members learn to relinquish responsibility for the individual's drinking. Point out that family involvement in rehabilitation can reduce family tensions.
• Refer adult children of alcoholics to the National Association for Children of Alcoholics.

Psychoactive drug abuse and dependence

The National Institute on Drug Abuse defines this condition as the use of a legal or an illegal drug that causes physical, mental, emotional, or social harm. Examples of abused drugs include narcotics, stimulants, depressants, antianxiety agents, and hallucinogens. Chronic drug abuse, especially I.V. use, can lead to life-threatening complications, such as cardiac and respiratory arrest, intracranial hemorrhage, acquired immunodeficiency syndrome, tetanus, subacute infective endocarditis, hepatitis, vasculitis, septicemia, thrombophlebitis, pulmonary emboli, gangrene, malaria, malnutrition and GI disturbances, respiratory infections, musculoskeletal dysfunction, trauma, depression, increased risk of suicide, and psychosis. Materials used to "cut" street drugs also can cause toxic or allergic reactions. (See *Understanding commonly abused substances,* pages 40 to 44.)

Psychoactive drug abuse can occur at any age. Experimentation with drugs commonly begins in adolescence or even earlier. Drug abuse often leads to addiction, which may involve physical or psychological dependence, or both. The most dangerous form of abuse occurs when users mix several drugs simultaneously—including alcohol.

Causes

Psychoactive drug abuse commonly results from a combination of low self-esteem, peer pressure, inadequate coping skills, and curiosity. Most people who are predisposed to drug abuse have few mental or emotional resources against stress, an excessive dependence on others, and a low tolerance for frustration. Taking the drug gives them pleasure by relieving

(Text continues on page 44.)

Understanding commonly abused substances

SUBSTANCE	SIGNS AND SYMPTOMS	INTERVENTIONS
Stimulants		
Cocaine • *Street names:* coke, flake, snow, nose candy, hits, crack (hardened form), rock, crank • *Routes:* ingestion, injection, sniffing, smoking • *Dependence:* psychological • *Duration of effect:* 15 minutes to 2 hours; with crack, rapid high of short duration followed by let-down feeling • *Medical uses:* local anesthetic	• *Of use:* abdominal pain; alternating euphoria and fear; anorexia; cardiotoxicity, such as ventricular fibrillation or cardiac arrest; coma; confusion; diaphoresis; dilated pupils; excitability; fever; grandiosity; hyperpnea; hypotension or hypertension; insomnia; irritability; nausea and vomiting; pallor or cyanosis; perforated nasal septum with prolonged use; pressured speech; psychotic behavior with large doses; respiratory arrest; seizures; spasms; tachycardia; tachypnea; visual, auditory, and olfactory hallucinations; weight loss • *Of withdrawal:* anxiety, depression, fatigue	• Place the patient in a quiet room. • If cocaine was ingested, induce vomiting or perform gastric lavage. Follow with activated charcoal and a saline cathartic. • If cocaine was sniffed, remove residual drug from mucous membranes. • Monitor vital signs. • Give propranolol for tachycardia. • Perform cardiopulmonary resuscitation for ventricular fibrillation and cardiac arrest as indicated. • Give a tepid sponge bath for fever. • Administer an anticonvulsant for seizures.
Amphetamines • *Street names:* for amphetamine sulfate — bennies, cartwheels, grennies; for methamphetamine — speed, meth, crystal; for dextroamphetamine sulfate — dexies, hearts, oranges • *Routes:* ingestion, injection • *Dependence:* psychological • *Duration of effect:* 1 to 4 hours • *Medical uses:* hyperkinesis, narcolepsy, weight control	• *Of use:* altered mental status (from confusion to paranoia), coma, diaphoresis, dilated reactive pupils, dry mouth, exhaustion, hallucinations, hyperactive deep tendon reflexes, hypertension, hyperthermia, paradoxical reaction in children, psychotic behavior with prolonged use, seizures, shallow respirations, tachycardia, tremors • *Of withdrawal:* abdominal tenderness, apathy, depression, disorientation, irritability, long periods of sleep, muscle aches, suicide (with sudden withdrawal)	• Place the patient in a quiet room. • If the drug was ingested, induce vomiting or perform gastric lavage; give activated charcoal and a saline or magnesium sulfate cathartic. • Add ammonium chloride or ascorbic acid to I.V. solution to acidify urine to a pH of 5. Also, administer mannitol to induce diuresis if needed. • Monitor vital signs. • Adminster a short-acting barbiturate, such as pentobarbital, for seizures; haloperidol for assaultive behavior; phentolamine for hypertension; propranolol for tachyarrhythmias; and lidocaine for ventricular arrhythmias. • Restrain the patient if he's experiencing hallucinations or paranoia. • Give a tepid sponge bath for fever. • Institute suicide precautions.

Understanding commonly abused substances *(continued)*

SUBSTANCE	SIGNS AND SYMPTOMS	INTERVENTIONS

Hallucinogens

SUBSTANCE	SIGNS AND SYMPTOMS	INTERVENTIONS
Lysergic acid diethylamide (LSD) • *Street names:* acid, microdot, sugar, big D • *Routes:* ingestion, smoking • *Dependence:* possibly psychological • *Duration of effect:* 8 to 12 hours • *Medical uses:* none	• *Of use:* abdominal cramps, arrhythmias, chills, depersonalization, diaphoresis, diarrhea, distorted visual perception and perception of time and space, dizziness, dry mouth, fever, grandiosity, hallucinations, heightened sense of awareness, hyperpnea, hypertension, illusions, increased salivation, muscle aches, mystical experiences, nausea, palpitations, seizures, tachycardia, vomiting • *Of withdrawal:* none	• Place the patient in a quiet room. • If the drug was ingested, induce vomiting or perform gastric lavage. Follow with activated charcoal and a cathartic. • Monitor vital signs, and give diazepam for seizures. • Reorient the patient to time, place, and person, and restrain him as necessary.
Phencyclidine • *Street names:* PCP, hog, angel dust, peace pill, crystal superjoint, elephant tranquilizer, rocket fuel • *Routes:* ingestion, injection, smoking • *Dependence:* possibly psychological • *Duration of effect:* 30 minutes to several days • *Medical uses:* veterinary anesthetic	• *Of use:* amnesia; blank stare; cardiac arrest; decreased awareness of surroundings; delusions; distorted body image; distorted sense of sight, hearing, and touch; drooling; euphoria; excitation and psychoses; fever; gait ataxia; hallucinations; hyperactivity; hypertensive crisis; individualized unpredictable effects; muscle rigidity; nystagmus; panic; poor perception of time and distance; possible chromosomal damage; psychotic behavior; recurrent coma; renal failure; seizures; sudden behavioral changes; tachycardia; violent behavior • *Of withdrawal:* none	• Place the patient in a quiet room. • If the drug was ingested, induce vomiting or perform gastric lavage. Follow with activated charcoal. • Add ascorbic acid to I.V. solution to acidify urine. • Monitor vital signs and urine output. • If needed, give a diuretic; propranolol for hypertension or tachycardia; nitroprusside for severe hypertensive crisis; diazepam for seizures; diazepam or haloperidol for agitation or psychotic behavior; and physostigmine salicylate, diazepam, chlordiazepoxide, or chlorpromazine for a "bad trip."

Depressants

SUBSTANCE	SIGNS AND SYMPTOMS	INTERVENTIONS
Alcohol • *Found in:* beer, wine, distilled spirits; also contained in cough syrup, after-shave, and mouthwash • *Route:* ingestion • *Dependence:* physical, psychological	• *Of acute use:* coma, decreased inhibitions, euphoria followed by depression or hostility, impaired judgment, incoordination, respiratory depression, slurred speech, unconsciousness, vomiting • *Of withdrawal:* delirium, hallucinations, seizures, tremors	• Place the patient in a quiet room. • If alcohol was ingested within 4 hours, induce vomiting or perform gastric lavage; give activated charcoal and a saline cathartic. • Monitor vital signs. *(continued)*

Understanding commonly abused substances (continued)

SUBSTANCE	SIGNS AND SYMPTOMS	INTERVENTIONS
Depressants (continued)		
Alcohol (continued) • *Duration of effect:* varies according to individual and amount ingested; metabolized at rate of 10 ml/hour • *Medical uses:* neurolysis (absolute alcohol); emergency tocolytic; treatment of ethylene glycol and methanol poisoning		• Administer diazepam for seizures and chlordiazepoxide, chloral hydrate, or paraldehyde for hallucinations and delirium. • Institute seizure precautions. • Provide I.V. fluid replacement as well as dextrose, thiamine, B-complex vitamins, and vitamin C to treat dehydration, hypoglycemia, and nutritional deficiencies. • Assess for aspiration pneumonia. • Prepare the patient for dialysis if his vital functions are severely depressed.
Benzodiazepines alprazolam, chlordiazepoxide, clonazepam, clorazepate, diazepam, flurazepam, halazepam, lorazepam, midazolam, oxazepam, prazepam, quazepam, temazepam, triazolam • *Street names:* dolls, green and whites, roaches, yellow jackets • *Routes:* ingestion, injection • *Dependence:* physical, psychological • *Duration of effect:* 4 to 8 hours • *Medical uses:* antianxiety agent, anticonvulsant, sedative, hypnotic	• *Of use:* ataxia, drowsiness, hypotension, increased self-confidence, relaxation, slurred speech • *Of overdose:* confusion, coma, drowsiness, respiratory depression • *Of withdrawal:* abdominal cramps, agitation, anxiety, diaphoresis, hypertension, tachycardia, tonic-clonic seizures, tremors, vomiting	• If the drug was ingested, induce vomiting or perform gastric lavage. Follow with activated charcoal and a cathartic. • Monitor the patient's vital signs. • Give supplemental oxygen for hypoxia-induced seizures. • Give I.V. fluids for hypertension and physostigmine salicylate for respiratory or central nervous system (CNS) depression.
Barbiturates amobarbital, phenobarbital, secobarbital • *Street names:* for barbiturates — downers, barbs; for amobarbital — blue angels, blue devils; for phenobarbital — purple hearts, goofballs; for secobarbital — reds, red devils	• *Of use:* absent reflexes, blisters or bullous lesions, cyanosis, depressed level of consciousness (LOC) — from confusion to coma, fever, flaccid muscles, hypotension, hypothermia, nystagmus, paradoxical reaction in children and elderly people, poor pupil reaction to light, respiratory depression	• If ingestion was recent, induce vomiting or perform gastric lavage. Follow with activated charcoal. • Monitor vital signs and perform frequent neurologic assessments. • Give an I.V. fluid bolus for hypotension and alkalinize urine.

Understanding commonly abused substances *(continued)*

SUBSTANCE	SIGNS AND SYMPTOMS	INTERVENTIONS
Depressants *(continued)*		
Barbiturates *(continued)* • *Routes:* ingestion, injection • *Dependence:* physical, psychological • *Duration:* 1 to 16 hours • *Medical uses:* anesthetic, anticonvulsant, sedative, hypnotic	• *Of withdrawal:* agitation, anxiety, fever, insomnia, orthostatic hypotension, tachycardia, tremors • *Of rapid withdrawal:* anorexia, apprehension, hallucinations, orthostatic hypotension, tonic-clonic seizures, tremors, weakness	• Use seizure precautions; relieve withdrawal symptoms. • Use a hypothermia or hyperthermia blanket for temperature alterations.
Opiates codeine, heroin, morphine, meperidine, opium • *Street names:* for heroin—junk, horse, H, smack; for morphine—morph, M • *Routes:* for codeine, meperidine, morphine—ingestion, injection, smoking; for heroin—ingestion, injection, inhalation, smoking; for opium—ingestion, smoking • *Dependence:* physical, psychological • *Duration of effect:* 3 to 6 hours • *Medical uses:* for codeine—analgesic, antitussive; for heroin—none; for morphine, meperidine—analgesic; for opium—analgesic, antidiarrheal	• *Of use:* anorexia, arrhythmias, clammy skin, constipation, constricted pupils, decreased LOC, detachment from reality, drowsiness, euphoria, hypotension, impaired judgment, increased pigmentation over veins, lack of concern, lethargy, nausea, needle marks, respiratory depression, seizures, shallow or slow respirations, skin lesions or abscesses, slurred speech, swollen or perforated nasal mucosa, thrombotic veins, urine retention, vomiting • *Of withdrawal:* abdominal cramps, anorexia, chills, diaphoresis, dilated pupils, hyperactive bowel sounds, irritability, nausea, panic, piloerection, runny nose, sweating, tremors, watery eyes, yawning	• If the drug was ingested, induce vomiting or perform gastric lavage. • Give naloxone until CNS effects are reversed. • Give I.V. fluids to increase circulatory volume. • Use extra blankets for hypothermia; if ineffective, use a hyperthermia blanket. • Reorient the patient to time, place, and person. • Assess breath sounds to monitor for pulmonary edema. • Monitor for signs and symptoms of withdrawal.
Cannabinoids		
Marijuana • *Street names:* pot, grass, weed, Mary Jane, roach, reefer, joint, THC • *Routes:* ingestion, smoking • *Dependence:* psychological	• *Of use:* acute psychosis; agitation; amotivational syndrome; anxiety; asthma; bronchitis; conjunctival reddening; decreased muscle strength; delusions; distorted sense of time and self-perception; dry mouth; euphoria; hallucinations; impaired cognition, short-	• Place the patient in a quiet room. • Monitor vital signs. • Give supplemental oxygen for respiratory depression and I.V. fluids for hypotension. • Give diazepam for extreme agitation and acute psychosis. *(continued)*

Understanding commonly abused substances *(continued)*

SUBSTANCE	SIGNS AND SYMPTOMS	INTERVENTIONS
Cannabinoids *(continued)*		
Marijuana *(continued)* • *Duration of effect:* 2 to 3 hours • *Medical uses:* antiemetic for chemotherapy	term memory, and mood; incoordination; increased hunger; increased systolic pressure when supine; orthostatic hypotension; paranoia; spontaneous laughter; tachycardia; vivid visual imagery • *Of withdrawal:* chills, decreased appetite, increased rapid-eye-movement sleep, insomnia, irritability, nervousness, restlessness, tremors, weight loss	

tension, abolishing loneliness, achieving a temporarily peaceful or euphoric state, or simply relieving boredom.

Drug dependence may follow experimentation with drugs in response to peer pressure. It also may follow the use of drugs to relieve physical pain, but this is an uncommon cause of drug dependence.

Signs and symptoms

The signs and symptoms of acute intoxication vary, depending on the drug. The drug user seldom seeks treatment specifically for his drug problem. Instead, he may seek emergency treatment for drug-related injuries or complications, such as a motor vehicle accident, burns from freebasing, an overdose, physical deterioration from illness or malnutrition, or withdrawal. Friends, family members, or law enforcement officials may bring the patient to the hospital because of respiratory depression, unconsciousness, acute injury, or a psychiatric crisis.

Examine the patient for signs and symptoms of drug use or drug-related complications as well as for clues to the type of drug ingested. For example, fever can result from stimulant or hallucinogen intoxication, from withdrawal, or from infection from I.V. drug use.

Inspect the eyes for lacrimation from opiate withdrawal, nystagmus from central nervous system (CNS) depressants or phencyclidine (PCP) intoxication, and drooping eyelids from opiate or CNS depressant use. Constricted pupils occur with opiate use or withdrawal; dilated pupils, with the use of hallucinogens or amphetamines.

Examine the nose for rhinorrhea from opiate withdrawal and the oral and nasal mucosa for signs of drug-induced irritation. Drug sniffing can result in inflammation, atrophy, or perforation of the nasal mucosa. Dental conditions commonly result from the poor oral hygiene associated with chronic drug use. Also inspect under the tongue for evidence of I.V. drug injection.

Inspect the patient's skin. Sweating, a common sign of intoxication with opiates or CNS stimulants, also accompanies most drug withdrawal syndromes. Drug use may induce a sensation of bugs crawling on the skin, known as formication; as a result, the patient's skin may be excoriated from scratching.

Needle marks or tracks are an obvious sign of I.V. drug abuse. Note that the patient may attempt to conceal or disguise injection sites with tattoos or by selecting an inconspicuous site, such as under the nails. In addition, self-injection can sometimes cause cellulitis or abscesses, especially in patients who also are chronic alcoholics. Puffy hands can be a late sign of thrombophlebitis or of fascial infection due to self-injection on the hands or arms.

Auscultation may disclose bilateral crackles and rhonchi caused by smoking and inhaling drugs or by opiate overdose. Other cardiopulmonary signs of overdose include pulmonary edema, respiratory depression, aspiration pneumonia, and hypotension. CNS stimulants and some hallucinogens may precipitate refractory acute-onset hypertension or cardiac arrhythmias. Withdrawal from opiates or depressants also can provoke arrhythmias and, occasionally, hypotension.

During opiate withdrawal, the patient may report abdominal pain, nausea, or vomiting. Opiate abusers also commonly complain of hemorrhoids, a consequence of the constipating effects of these drugs. When examining the patient, palpation of an enlarged liver, with or without tenderness, may indicate hepatitis.

Neurologic symptoms of drug abuse include tremors, hyperreflexia, hyporeflexia, and seizures. Abrupt withdrawal may precipitate signs of CNS depression ranging from lethargy to coma, hallucinations, or signs of overstimulation, including euphoria and violent behavior.

Carefully review the patient's medical history. Suspect drug abuse if he reports a painful injury or chronic illness but refuses a diagnostic workup. In his attempt to obtain drugs, the dependent patient may feign illnesses, such as migraine headaches, myocardial infarction, and renal colic; claim an allergy to over-the-counter analgesics; or even request a specific medication. Also be alert for a previous history of overdose or a high tolerance for potentially addictive drugs. I.V. drug users may have a history of hepatitis or human immunodeficiency virus (HIV) infection from often sharing dirty needles. Female drug users may report a history of amenorrhea.

A patient who abuses drugs may give a fictitious name and address. He may be reluctant to discuss previous hospitalizations or may seek treatment at a medical facility across town rather than in his own neighborhood. If possible, interview the patient's family members to verify his history responses.

If the patient admits to drug use, try to determine the extent to which this behavior interferes with his normal functioning. Note whether he expresses a desire to overcome his dependence on drugs. If possible, obtain a drug history consisting of substances ingested, amount, frequency, and last dose. Expect incomplete or inaccurate responses. Drug-induced amnesia, a depressed level of consciousness, or ignorance may distort the patient's recollection of the facts; he also may deliberately fabricate answers to avoid arrest or to conceal a suicide attempt.

The hospitalized drug abuser is likely to be uncooperative, disruptive, or even violent. He may experience mood swings, anxiety, impaired memory, sleep disturbances, flashbacks, slurred speech, depression, and thought disorders. Some patients resort to plays on sympathy, bribery, or threats to obtain drugs or try to manipulate caregivers by pitting one against another.

Diagnosis

For characteristic findings in patients with this condition, see *Diagnosing substance dependence and related disorders,* page 35. Various tests can confirm drug use, determine the amount and type of drug taken, and reveal complications. For example, a serum or urine drug screen can detect recently ingested substances.

Characteristic findings in other tests include elevated serum globulin levels, hypoglycemia, leukocytosis, liver function abnormalities, positive Venereal Disease Research Laboratory (VDRL) or rapid plasma reagin test results due to elevated protein fractions, elevated mean corpuscular hemoglobin levels, elevated uric acid levels, and reduced blood urea nitrogen levels.

Treatment

The patient with acute drug intoxication should receive symptomatic treatment based on the drug ingested. Measures include fluid replacement therapy and nutritional and vitamin supplements, if indicated; detoxification with the same drug or a pharmacologically similar drug (exceptions include cocaine, hallucinogens, and marijuana, which are not used for detoxification); sedatives to induce sleep; anticholinergics and antidiarrheal agents to relieve GI distress; antianxiety drugs for severe agitation, especially in cocaine abusers; and symptomatic treatment of complications. Depending on the dosage and time elapsed before admission, additional treatment may include gastric lavage, induced emesis, activated charcoal, forced diuresis and, possibly, hemoperfusion or hemodialysis.

Treatment of drug dependence commonly involves a triad of care: detoxification, short- and long-term rehabilitation, and aftercare; the latter means a lifetime of abstinence, usually aided by participation in Narcotics Anonymous or a similar self-help group.

Detoxification, the controlled and gradual withdrawal of an abused drug, is achieved through substitution of a drug with similar action. Such gradual replacement of the abused drug with the substitute drug controls the effects of withdrawal, thus reducing the patient's discomfort and associated risks.

Depending on which drug the patient has abused, detoxification may be managed on an inpatient or outpatient basis. For example, withdrawal from depressants can produce hazardous effects, such as generalized tonic-clonic seizures, status epilepticus, and hypotension; the severity of these effects determines whether the patient can be safely treated as an outpatient or requires hospitalization.

Withdrawal from depressants usually doesn't require detoxification. Opioid withdrawal causes severe physical discomfort and can even be life-threatening. To minimize these effects, chronic opioid abusers commonly are detoxified with methadone.

To ease withdrawal from opioids, depressants, and other drugs, useful nonchemical measures may include psychotherapy, exercise, relaxation techniques, and nutritional support. Sedatives and tranquilizers may be administered temporarily to help the patient cope with insomnia, anxiety, and depression.

After withdrawal, rehabilitation is needed to prevent recurrence of drug abuse. Rehabilitation programs are available for both inpatients and outpatients. These programs usually last a month or longer and may include individual, group, and family psychotherapy. During and after rehabilitation, participation in a drug-oriented self-help group may also be helpful. The largest of these groups is Narcotics Anonymous.

Special considerations

• Focus on restoring physical health, educating the patient and his family about drug abuse and dependence, providing support, and encouraging participation in drug treatment programs and self-help groups.

During an acute episode

• Continuously monitor the patient's vital signs, and observe for complications of overdose and withdrawal, such as cardiopulmonary arrest, seizures, and aspiration.
• Based on standard hospital policy, you should institute appropriate measures to help prevent possible suicide attempts by the patient.
• Give medications to decrease withdrawal symptoms; monitor and record their effectiveness.
• Try to maintain a quiet, safe environment during withdrawal from any drug because excessive noise may agitate the patient.
• Make sure that you remove any harmful objects from the patient's room.
• Use restraints only if you suspect that the patient might harm himself or others.
• Institute seizure precautions.

After the acute episode

- Learn to control your emotional response to the patient's undesirable behaviors, which commonly include psychological dependency, manipulation, anger, frustration, and alienation.
- Set appropriate limits for dealing with demanding, manipulative behavior.
- Promote adequate nutrition and monitor the patient's nutritional intake.
- Administer medications carefully to prevent hoarding by the patient. Remember to check the patient's mouth to ensure that he has swallowed the medication.
- Closely monitor any visitors who might supply the patient with drugs.
- Refer the patient for detoxification and rehabilitation as appropriate. Make sure that you provide him with a list of available resources.
- Encourage family members to seek help whether or not the abuser seeks it. You can suggest private therapy or community mental health clinics.
- If the patient refuses to participate in a rehabilitation program, teach him how to minimize the risk of drug-related complications.
- Review measures for preventing HIV infection and hepatitis. Stress that these infections are readily transmitted by sharing needles with other drug users and by unprotected sexual intercourse.
- Advise the patient to use a new needle for every drug injection or to clean the needles with a solution of chlorine bleach and water.
- Emphasize the importance of using a condom during intercourse to prevent disease transmission and pregnancy. If necessary, teach the female drug abuser about other methods of birth control.
- Explain the devastating effects of drugs on the developing fetus.

Self-test questions

You can quickly review your comprehension of this chapter on psychoactive substance abuse, alcoholism, and drug abuse by answering the following questions. The correct answers to these questions and their rationales appear on pages 156 and 157.

1. Substance intoxication is characterized by:
   a. development of a reversible substance-specific syndrome due to recent ingestion of, or exposure to, a substance.
   b. continued use of a substance despite having persistent or recurrent social or interpersonal problems that are caused or exacerbated by the effects of the substance.
   c. spending a great deal of time in activities necessary to obtain the substance, use the substance, or recover from its effects.
   d. the need for increased amounts of the substance to achieve the desired effect.

Case history questions

Paul Gibson, a 26-year-old with an alcoholic father, has been drinking heavily in response to increasing stress, peer pressure, and the social approval and easy availability of alcohol when he is among his friends.

2. What part is the father's alcoholism apt to play in Paul's situation?
   a. A child's propensity for alcoholism is not related to his parents'.
   b. Parental alcoholism ensures that children have at least a 50% chance of becoming alcoholics themselves.
   c. An offspring of one alcoholic parent is seven to eight times more likely to become alcoholic.
   d. Both parents would have to be alcoholics for the offspring to develop alcohol addiction.

3. Evaluating Paul for alcoholism may be difficult because he:
  a. has not experienced blackouts.
  b. is not violent when intoxicated.
  c. demonstrates no untreated injuries.
  d. is currently able to maintain a functional life.

4. Paul says he can do without alcohol whenever he wishes, and embarks on a period of abstinence. Early signs of alcohol withdrawal to watch for include:
  a. severe tremulousness and agitation.
  b. hallucinations and violent behavior.
  c. anxiety, insomnia, and diaphoresis.
  d. major motor seizures.

5. Paul begins to drink again after a particularly hard day at work. On his way home, he's stopped by the highway patrol for erratic driving and is tested for intoxication. The accepted level for intoxication is:
  a. 0.05% weight volume (100 mg/dl).
  b. 0.075% weight volume (150 mg/dl).
  c. 0.10% weight volume (200 mg/dl).
  d. 0.20% weight volume (400 mg/dl).

6. When Paul realizes that total abstinence from alcohol is the only effective treatment, he's referred to Alcoholics Anonymous, and the doctor starts him on aversion therapy using:
  a. diazepam.
  b. disulfiram.
  c. promazine.
  d. prochlorperazine.

Johanna Gutschow, a 33-year-old homeless woman, is dropped off at the emergency department by friends who fear that she may have overdosed on "smack." She is unconscious and sweating. Serum and urine drug screens for opiates are carried out.

7. Which of the following signs would you expect to find on physical examination?

a. hypertension and cardiac arrhythmias.
b. dilated pupils.
c. perforation of the nasal septum mucosa.
d. constricted pupils.

8. Johanna will require supportive therapy that's based on her symptoms. In addition, she will require detoxification using:

a. naloxone.
b. methadone.
c. an antianxiety agent.
d. an anticholinergic.

CHAPTER 4

Schizophrenic Disorders

Characterized by disordered thinking, schizophrenic disorders include schizophrenia and delusional disorders.

Schizophrenia

This disorder is characterized by disturbances (for at least 6 months) in thought content and form, perception, affect, sense of self, volition, interpersonal relationships, and psychomotor behavior. The *Diagnostic and Statistical Manual of Mental Disorders,* 4th edition *(DSM-IV),* recognizes paranoid, disorganized, catatonic, undifferentiated, and residual schizophrenia. Schizophrenia affects 1% to 2% of the U.S. population and is equally prevalent in both sexes. Onset of symptoms usually occurs during adolescence or early adulthood. The disorder produces varying degrees of impairment. Up to one-third of patients with schizophrenia have just one psychotic episode and no more. Some patients have no disability between periods of exacerbation; others need continuous institutional care. The prognosis worsens with each episode.

Causes

Schizophrenia may result from a combination of genetic, biological, cultural, and psychological factors. Some evidence supports a genetic predisposition. Close relatives of persons with schizophrenia are up to 50 times more likely to develop schizophrenia; the closer the degree of biological relatedness, the higher the risk.

The most widely accepted biochemical hypothesis holds that schizophrenia results from excessive activity at dopaminergic synapses. Other neurotransmitter alterations may also contribute to schizophrenic symptoms. In addition, patients with schizophrenia have structural abnormalities of the frontal and temporolimbic systems.

Numerous psychological and sociocultural causes, such as disturbed family and interpersonal patterns, also have been proposed. Schizophrenia has a higher incidence among lower socioeconomic groups, possibly related to downward social drift, lack of upward socioeconomic mobility, and high stress levels that may stem from poverty, social failure, illness, and inadequate social resources. Higher incidence also is linked to low birth weight and congenital deafness.

Signs and symptoms

Schizophrenia is associated with a variety of abnormal behaviors; therefore, signs and symptoms vary widely, depending on the type and phase (prodromal, active, or residual) of the illness. (See *Phases of schizophrenia.*)

Behaviors and functional deficiencies can vary. Watch for these key signs and symptoms:
• ambivalence—coexisting strong positive and negative feelings, leading to emotional conflict
• apathy
• clang associations—words that rhyme or sound alike used in an illogical, nonsensical manner, for instance, "It's the rain, train, pain."
• concrete associations—inability to form or understand abstract thoughts
• delusions—false ideas or beliefs accepted as real by the patient. Delusions of grandeur, persecution, and reference (distorted belief regarding the relation between events and one's self, for example, a belief that television programs address the patient on a personal level) are common in schizophrenia. Also common are feelings of being controlled, somatic illness, and depersonalization.
• echolalia—meaningless repetition of words or phrases
• echopraxia—involuntary repetition of movements observed in others
• flight of ideas—rapid succession of incomplete and unconnected ideas
• hallucinations—false sensory perceptions with no basis in reality. Usually visual or auditory, hallucinations also may be olfactory (smell), gustatory (taste), or tactile (touch).

Phases of schizophrenia

Schizophrenia usually occurs in three phases: prodromal, active, and residual.

Prodromal phase

The *DSM-IV* characterizes the prodromal phase as clear deterioration in functioning before the active phase of the disturbance that is not due to a disturbance in mood or to a psychoactive substance use disorder and that involves at least two of the following signs and symptoms:

• marked social isolation or withdrawal
• marked impairment in role functioning as wage-earner, student, or homemaker
• markedly peculiar behavior
• marked impairment in personal hygiene and grooming
• blunted or inappropriate affect
• digressive, vague, overelaborate, or circumstantial speech, or poverty of speech, or poverty of content of speech
• odd beliefs or magical thinking that influences behavior and is inconsistent with cultural norms
• unusual perceptual experiences
• marked lack of initiative, interests, or energy.

Family members or friends may report personality changes. Typically insidious, this phase may extend over several months or years.

Active phase

During the active phase, the patient exhibits frankly psychotic symptoms. Psychiatric evaluation may reveal delusions, hallucinations, loosening of associations, incoherence, and catatonic behavior. The patient's psychosocial history may also disclose a particular stressor before the onset of this phase.

Residual phase

According to the *DSM-IV,* the residual phase follows the active phase and occurs when at least two of the symptoms noted in the prodromal phase persist. These symptoms do not result from a disturbance in mood or from a psychoactive substance use disorder.

The residual phase resembles the prodromal phase, except that disturbances in affect and role functioning usually are more severe. Delusions and hallucinations may persist.

• illusions – false sensory perceptions with some basis in reality, for example, a car's backfiring mistaken for a gunshot
• loose associations – rapid shifts among unrelated ideas
• magical thinking – belief that thoughts or wishes can control other people or events
• neologisms – bizarre words that have meaning only for the patient
• poor interpersonal relationships
• regression – return to an earlier developmental stage
• thought blocking – sudden interruption in the patient's train of thought
• withdrawal – disinterest in objects, people, or surroundings

• word salad—illogical word groupings, for example, "She had a star, barn, plant."

Diagnosis

After complete physical and psychiatric examinations rule out an organic cause of symptoms, such as an amphetamine-induced psychosis, a diagnosis of schizophrenia is made if the patient's symptoms match those put forth in the *DSM-IV*. For characteristic findings, see *Diagnosing schizophrenia.*

Treatment

In schizophrenia, treatment focuses on meeting the physical and psychosocial needs of the patient, based on his previous level of adjustment and his response to medical and nursing interventions. Treatment typically includes a combination of drug therapy, long-term psychotherapy for the patient and his family, psychosocial rehabilitation, vocational counseling, and the use of community resources.

The primary treatment for more than 30 years, antipsychotic drugs (sometimes called neuroleptic drugs) appear to work by blocking postsynaptic dopamine receptors. These drugs reduce the incidence of psychotic symptoms, such as hallucinations and delusions, and relieve anxiety and agitation. Other psychiatric drugs, such as antidepressants and anxiolytics, may be prescribed to control associated signs and symptoms.

Some antipsychotic drugs are associated with numerous adverse reactions, several of which are irreversible. Most experts agree that patients who are withdrawn, isolated, or apathetic show little improvement after this drug treatment. (See *Reviewing adverse effects of antipsychotic drugs,* page 58.)

High-potency antipsychotics include fluphenazine, haloperidol, thiothixene, and trifluoperazine. Loxapine, molindone, and perphenazine are intermediate in potency, and chlorpromazine and thioridazine are low-potency agents. Haloperidol decanoate, fluphenazine decanoate, and fluphenazine enanthate are depot formulations that are implanted I.M.; this method allows a gradual release of the drug over a 30-day period, thus improving compliance. A new antipsychotic, risperidone, also is reported to be effective.

Clozapine, which differs chemically from other antipsychotic drugs, may be prescribed for severely ill patients who fail to respond to standard treatment. This agent effectively

Diagnosing schizophrenia

The American Psychiatric Association uses the following criteria to diagnose a person with schizophrenia.

Characteristic symptoms

A person with schizophrenia has two or more of the following symptoms (each present for a significant time during a 1-month period—or less if successfully treated):

• delusions
• hallucinations
• disorganized speech
• grossly disorganized or catatonic behavior
• negative symptoms.

The diagnosis requires only one of these characteristic symptoms if the person's delusions are bizarre or if hallucinations consist of a voice issuing a running commentary on the person's behavior or thoughts, or two or more voices conversing.

Social and occupational dysfunction

For a significant period beginning with the onset of the disturbance, one or more major areas of functioning (such as work, interpersonal relations, or self-care) are markedly below the level achieved before the onset.

When the disturbance begins in childhood or adolescence, the dysfunction takes the form of failure to achieve the expected level of interpersonal, academic, or occupational development.

Duration

Continuous signs of the disturbance persist for at least 6 months. The 6-month period must include at least 1 month of symptoms (or less if signs and symptoms have been successfully treated) that match the characteristic symptoms and may include periods of prodromal or residual symptoms.

During the prodromal or residual periods, signs of the disturbance may be manifested by only negative symptoms or by two or more characteristic symptoms in a less severe form.

Exclusions

Schizoaffective disorder and mood disorder with psychotic features have been ruled out for these reasons: either no major depressive, manic, or mixed episodes have occurred concurrently with the active-phase symptoms *or* if mood episodes have occurred during active-phase symptoms, their total duration has been brief relative to the duration of the active and residual periods.

The disturbance is not due to the direct physiologic effects of a substance or a general medical condition.

Relationship to a pervasive developmental disorder

If the person has a history of autistic disorder or another pervasive developmental disorder, the additional diagnosis of schizophrenia is appropriate only if prominent delusions or hallucinations also are present for at least 1 month (or less if successfully treated).

Reviewing adverse effects of antipsychotic drugs

Antipsychotic drugs (sometimes known as neuroleptic drugs) can cause sedative, anticholinergic, or extrapyramidal effects; orthostatic hypotension; and, rarely, neuroleptic malignant syndrome.

Sedative, anticholinergic, and extrapyramidal effects

High-potency drugs (such as haloperidol) are minimally sedative and minimally anticholinergic but result in a high incidence of extrapyramidal adverse effects. Intermediate-potency agents (such as molindone) are associated with a moderate incidence of adverse effects, whereas low-potency drugs (such as chlorpromazine) are highly sedative and anticholinergic but elicit few extrapyramidal adverse effects.

The most common extrapyramidal effects are dystonia, parkinsonism, tardive dyskinesia, and akathisia. Dystonia most frequently occurs in young male patients, usually within the first few days of treatment. Characterized by severe tonic contractions of the muscles in the neck, mouth, and tongue, dystonia may be misdiagnosed as a psychotic symptom. Diphenhydramine or benztropine administered I.M. or I.V. provides rapid relief.

Drug-induced parkinsonism results in bradykinesia, muscle rigidity, shuffling or propulsive gait, stooped posture, flat facial affect, tremors, and drooling. Parkinsonism may occur from 1 week to several months after the initiation of drug treatment. Drugs prescribed to reverse or prevent this syndrome include benztropine, trihexyphenidyl, and amantadine.

Tardive dyskinesia can occur after only 6 months of continuous therapy and is usually irreversible. No effective treatment is available for this disorder, which is characterized by various involuntary movements of the mouth and jaw; flapping or writhing; purposeless, rapid, and jerky movements of the arms and legs; and dystonic posture of the neck and trunk.

Signs and symptoms of akathisia include restlessness, pacing, and an inability to rest or sit still. Propranolol relieves this adverse effect.

Orthostatic hypotension

Low-potency neuroleptics can cause orthostatic hypotension because they block alpha-adrenergic receptors. If hypotension is severe, place the patient in the supine position and give I.V. fluids for hypovolemia. If further treatment is necessary, an alpha-adrenergic agonist, such as norepinephrine or metaraminol, may be ordered to relieve hypotension. Mixed alpha- and beta-adrenergic drugs, such as epinephrine, or beta-adrenergic drugs, such as isoproterenol, should not be given because they can further reduce blood pressure.

Neuroleptic malignant syndrome

This life-threatening syndrome occurs in up to 1% of patients taking antipsychotic drugs. Signs and symtoms include fever, muscle rigidity, and altered level of consciousness occurring hours to months after initiating drug therapy or increasing the dose. Treatment is symptomatic, largely consisting of dantrolene and other measures to counter muscle rigidity associated with hyperthermia. You'll need to continuously monitor the patient's vital signs and mental status.

controls a wider range of psychotic signs and symptoms without the usual adverse effects. However, clozapine can cause drowsiness, sedation, excessive salivation, tachycardia, dizziness, and seizures as well as agranulocytosis, a potentially fatal blood disorder characterized by a low white blood cell count and pronounced neutropenia.

Routine blood monitoring is essential to detect the estimated 1% to 2% of all patients taking clozapine who develop agranulocytosis. If caught in the early stages, this disorder is reversible.

Clinicians disagree about the effectiveness of psychotherapy in schizophrenia. Some consider it to be a useful adjunct to drug therapy. Other studies suggest that psychosocial rehabilitation, education, and social skills training are more productive; in addition to improving their understanding of the disorder, these methods teach the patient and his family coping strategies, effective communication techniques, and social skills.

Special considerations

• Evaluate the patient's ability to carry out activities of daily living, paying special attention to his nutritional status. Monitor his weight if he isn't eating. If he thinks that his food is poisoned, let him fix his own food when possible, or offer foods in closed containers that he can open. If you give liquid medication in a unit-dose container, allow the patient to open the container.

• Maintain a safe environment, minimizing stimuli. Administer prescribed medications to decrease symptoms and anxiety. Use physical restraints according to your hospital's policy.

• Adopt an accepting and consistent approach with the patient. Short, repeated contacts are best until trust has been established.

• Avoid promoting dependence. Reward positive behavior to help the patient improve his level of functioning.

• Engage the patient in reality-oriented activities that involve human contact, such as inpatient social skills training groups, outpatient day care, and sheltered workshops. Provide reality-based explanations for distorted body images or hypochondriacal complaints. Explain to the patient that his private language, autistic inventions, or neologisms, are not understood. Set limits on inappropriate behavior.

• If the patient is hallucinating, explore the content of the hallucinations. If he hears voices, find out if he believes that he must do what they command. Explore the emotions connected with the hallucinations but don't argue about them. If possible, change the subject.

• Teach the patient techniques that interrupt the hallucinations (listening to an audiocassette player, singing out loud, or reading out loud).

• Don't tease or joke with a schizophrenic patient. Choose words and phrases that are unambiguous and clearly understood. For instance, a patient who's told "That procedure will be done on the floor" may become frightened, thinking he'll need to lie down on the floor.

• If the patient expresses suicidal thoughts, take suicide precautions. Document his behavior and your precautions.

• If he's expressing homicidal thoughts (for example, "I have to kill my mother"), institute homicidal precautions. Notify the doctor and the potential victim. Document the patient's comments and who was notified.

• Don't touch the patient without telling him first exactly what you're going to do—for example, "I'm going to put this cuff on your arm so I can take your blood pressure." If necessary, postpone procedures that require physical contact with hospital personnel until he's less suspicious or agitated.

• Remember, institutionalization may produce symptoms and handicaps that are not part of the patient's illness, so evaluate symptoms carefully.

• Mobilize community resources to provide a support system for the patient. Ongoing support is essential to his mastery of social skills.

• Encourage compliance with the medication regimen to prevent a relapse. Also, monitor the patient carefully for adverse drug effects, including drug-induced parkinsonism, acute dystonia, akathisia, tardive dyskinesia, and malignant neuroleptic syndrome. Document such effects promptly.

• Help the patient explore possible connections between anxiety and stress and the exacerbation of symptoms.

For catatonic schizophrenia

• Evaluate the patient for physical illness. Remember that the mute patient won't complain of pain or physical symptoms; if he's in a bizarre posture, he's at risk for pressure ulcers or decreased circulation to a body area.

• Meet physical needs for adequate food, fluid, exercise, and elimination; follow orders with respect to nutrition, urinary catheterization, and enema.

• Provide range-of-motion exercises or help the patient ambulate every 2 hours.

• Prevent physical exhaustion and injury during periods of hyperactivity.

• Tell the patient directly and concisely what needs to be done. Don't offer the negativistic patient a choice. For example, you might say, "It's time to go for a walk. Let's go."

• Spend some time with the patient even if he's mute and unresponsive. The patient is acutely aware of his environment even though he seems not to be. Your presence can be reassuring and supportive.

• Verbalize for the patient the message his nonverbal behavior seems to convey; encourage him to do so as well.

• Offer reality orientation. You might say, "The leaves on the trees are turning colors and the air is cooler. It's fall!" Emphasize reality to reduce distorted perceptions.

• Stay alert for violent outbursts; get help promptly to intervene safely for yourself and the patient.

For paranoid schizophrenia

• When the patient is newly admitted, minimize his contact with the staff.

• Don't crowd the patient physically or psychologically; he may strike out to protect himself.

• Be flexible; allow the patient some control. Approach him in a calm and unhurried manner. Let him talk about anything he wishes initially, but keep conversation light and social, and avoid entering into power struggles.

• Respond to the patient's condescending attitudes (arrogance, sarcasm, or open hostility) with neutral remarks.

• Don't let the patient put you on the defensive and don't take his remarks personally. If he tells you to leave him alone, do leave but return soon. Brief contacts with the patient may be most useful at first.

• Don't try to combat the patient's delusions with logic. Instead, respond to feelings, themes, or underlying needs – for example, "It seems you feel you've been treated unfairly" (persecution).

• Be honest and dependable. Don't threaten or promise what you can't fulfill.

Delusional disorder or paranoid schizophrenia?

To distinguish between these two disorders, consider the following characteristics.

Delusional disorder
In a delusional disorder, the patient's delusions reflect reality and are arranged into a coherent system. They're based on misinterpretations of, or elaborations on, reality.

The patient doesn't experience hallucinations, and his affect and behavior are normal.

Paranoid schizophrenia
In paranoid schizophrenia, the patient's delusions are scattered, illogical, and incoherently arranged with no relation to reality.

The patient may have hallucinations, his affect is inappropriate and inconsistent, and his behavior is bizarre.

• If the patient is taking clozapine, stress the importance of returning weekly to the hospital or an outpatient setting to have his blood monitored.

• Teach the patient the importance of complying with the medication regimen. Tell him to report any adverse reactions instead of stopping the drug. If he takes a slow-release formulation, make sure he understands when to return for his next dose of medication.

• Involve the patient's family in his treatment. Teach them how to recognize an impending relapse and suggest ways to manage symptoms, such as tension, nervousness, insomnia, decreased concentration ability, and loss of interest.

Delusional disorders

According to the *DSM-IV*, delusional disorders are marked by false beliefs with a plausible basis in reality. Formerly referred to as paranoid disorders, delusional disorders involve erotomanic, grandiose, persecutory, or somatic themes. (For more information, see *Delusional disorder or paranoid schizophrenia?*) Some patients experience several types of delusions; others experience unspecified delusions with no dominant theme. (See *Delusional themes.*)

Delusional themes

In a patient with a delusional disorder, the delusions usually are well systematized and follow a predominant theme. Common delusional themes are listed below.

Erotomanic delusions

A prevalent delusional theme, erotomanic delusions concern romantic or spiritual love. The patient believes that he shares in an idealized (rather than sexual) relationship with someone of higher status—a superior at work, a celebrity, or an anonymous stranger.

The patient may hold this delusion in secret but more commonly will try to contact the object of his delusion through calls, letters, gifts, or even spying. He may attempt to rescue his beloved from imagined danger. The patient with erotomanic delusions frequently harasses public figures and often comes to the attention of the police.

Grandiose delusions

The patient with grandiose delusions believes that he has great, unrecognized talent, special insight, or prophetic power or has made an important discovery. To achieve recognition, he may contact government agencies, such as the Federal Bureau of Investigation. The patient with a religiously oriented delusion of grandeur may become a cult leader. Less commonly, he believes that he shares a special relationship with some well-known personality, such as a rock star or world leader. The patient may believe himself to be a famous person, his identity usurped by an imposter.

Jealous delusions

These delusions focus on infidelity. For example, a patient may insist that his spouse or lover has been unfaithful and may search for evidence to justify the delusion such as spots on bed sheets. He may confront his partner, try to control her movements, follow her, or track down her suspected lover. He may physically assault her or, less likely, his perceived rival.

Persecutory delusions

The patient suffering from persecutory delusions, the most common delusional theme, believes that he's being followed, harassed, plotted against, poisoned, mocked, or deliberately prevented from achieving his long-term goals. These delusions may evolve into a simple or complex persecution scheme, in which even the slightest injustice is interpreted as part of the scheme.

Such a patient may file numerous lawsuits or seek redress from government agencies (querulous paranoia). A patient who becomes resentful and angry may lash out violently against the alleged offender.

Somatic delusions

This delusional theme centers on an imagined physical defect or deformity. The patient may perceive a foul odor coming from his skin, mouth, rectum, or other body part. Other delusions involve skin-crawling insects, internal parasites, or physical illness.

Delusional disorders commonly begin in middle or late adulthood, usually between ages 40 and 55, but they can occur at a younger age. These uncommon illnesses affect less than 1% of the population; the incidence is about equal in men and women. Typically chronic, these disorders often interfere with social and marital relationships but seldom impair intellectual or occupational functioning significantly.

Causes

Delusional disorders of later life strongly suggest a hereditary predisposition. At least one study has linked the development of delusional disorders to inferiority feelings in the family. Some researchers suggest that delusional disorders are the product of specific early childhood experiences within an authoritarian family structure. Others hold that anyone with a sensitive personality is particularly vulnerable to developing a delusional disorder.

Certain medical conditions are known to exaggerate the risks of delusional disorders: head injury, chronic alcoholism, deafness, and aging. Predisposing factors linked to aging include isolation, lack of stimulating interpersonal relationships, physical illness, and diminished hearing and vision. Severe stress may also precipitate a delusional disorder.

Signs and symptoms

The psychiatric history of a delusional patient may be unremarkable, aside from behavior related to his delusions. He's likely to report problems with social and marital relationships. He may describe a life marked by social isolation or hostility but deny feeling lonely, relentlessly criticizing or placing unreasonable demands on others.

Gathering accurate information from a delusional patient may prove difficult. He may deny his feelings, disregard the circumstances leading to his hospitalization, and refuse treatment. However, the patient's responses and behavior during the interview provide clues that can help to identify his disorder, and family members may confirm your observations.

For example, note how effectively the patient communicates. He may be evasive or reluctant to answer questions. Alternatively, he may be overly talkative, explaining events in great detail and emphasizing what he has achieved, prominent people he knows, or places he has traveled. Statements

Diagnosing delusional disorders

In an individual with suspected delusional disorder, psychiatric examination confirms the diagnosis. The examiner bases the diagnosis on the following criteria set forth in the *DSM-IV:*

• Nonbizarre delusions of at least 1 month's duration are present, involving real-life situations, such as being followed, poisoned, infected, loved at a distance, or deceived by one's spouse or lover.

• The patient's symptoms have never met the criteria known as *characteristic symptoms* of schizophrenia. However, tactile and olfactory hallucinations may be present if they are related to a delusional theme.

• Apart from being affected by the delusion or its ramifications, the patient is not markedly impaired functionally nor is his behavior obviously odd or bizarre.

• If mood episodes have occurred concurrently with delusions, their total duration has been brief relative to the duration of the delusional disturbance.

• The disturbance is not due to the direct physiologic effects of a substance or a general medical condition.

that first seem logical may later prove irrelevant. Some of his answers may be contradictory, jumbled, or irrational.

Be alert for expressions of denial, projection, and rationalization. Once delusions become firmly entrenched, the patient will no longer seek to justify his beliefs. However, if he's still struggling to maintain his delusional defenses, he may make statements that reveal his condition, such as "People at work won't talk to me because I'm smarter than they." Accusatory statements are also characteristic of the patient with a delusional disorder. Record pervasive delusional themes (for example, grandiose or persecutory).

Also watch for nonverbal cues, such as excessive vigilance or obvious apprehension on entering the room. During questions, the patient may listen intently, reacting defensively to imagined slights or insults. He may sit at the edge of his seat or fold his arms as if to shield himself. If he carries papers or money, he may clutch them firmly.

Diagnosis

For characteristic findings in patients with this condition, see *Diagnosing delusional disorders.*

In addition, blood and urine tests, psychological tests, and neurologic evaluation can rule out organic causes of the delusions, such as amphetamine-induced psychoses and Alzheimer's disease. Endocrine function tests rule out hyperadrenalism, pernicious anemia, and thyroid disorders such as "myxedemic madness."

Treatment

Effective treatment of delusional disorders, consisting of a combination of drug therapy and psychotherapy, must correct the behavior and mood disturbances that result from the patient's mistaken belief system. Treatment also may include mobilizing a support system for the isolated elderly patient.

Drug treatment with antipsychotic agents is similar to that used in schizophrenic disorders. Antipsychotics appear to work by blocking postsynaptic dopamine receptors. These drugs reduce the incidence of psychotic symptoms, such as hallucinations and delusions, and relieve anxiety and agitation. Other psychiatric drugs, such as antidepressants and anxiolytics, may be prescribed to control associated symptoms.

High-potency antipsychotics include fluphenazine, haloperidol, thiothixene, and trifluoperazine. Loxapine, molindone, and perphenazine are intermediate in potency, and chlorpromazine and thioridazine are low-potency agents. Haloperidol decanoate, fluphenazine decanoate, and fluphenazine enanthate are depot formulations that are implanted I.M. and release the drug gradually over a 30-day period, improving compliance.

Clozapine, which differs chemically from other antipsychotic drugs, may be prescribed for severely ill patients who fail to respond to standard treatment. This agent effectively controls a wider range of psychotic symptoms without the usual adverse effects. However, clozapine can cause drowsiness, sedation, excessive salivation, tachycardia, dizziness, and seizures as well as agranulocytosis, a potentially fatal blood disorder characterized by a low white blood cell count and pronounced neutropenia. Routine blood monitoring is essential to detect the estimated 1% to 2% of all patients taking clozapine who develop agranulocytosis. If caught in the early stages, this disorder is reversible.

Special considerations

• In dealing with the delusional patient, be direct, straightforward, and dependable. Whenever possible, elicit his feedback. Move slowly in a matter-of-fact manner. Respond without anger or defensiveness to his hostile remarks.
• Respect the patient's privacy and space needs. Avoid touching him unnecessarily.

• Take steps to reduce social isolation, if the patient allows. Gradually increase social contacts after he has become comfortable with the staff.
• Watch for refusal of medication or food resulting from the patient's irrational fear of poisoning.
• Monitor the patient carefully for adverse effects of antipsychotic drugs, such as drug-induced parkinsonism, acute dystonia, akathisia, tardive dyskinesia, and malignant neuroleptic syndrome. If the patient is taking clozapine, stress the importance of returning weekly to the hospital or an outpatient setting to have his blood monitored.
• Involve the family in treatment. Teach them how to recognize an impending relapse, and suggest ways to manage symptoms. These include tension, nervousness, insomnia, decreased concentration ability, and apathy.

Self-test questions

You can quickly review your comprehension of this chapter on schizophrenic disorders by answering the following questions. The correct answers to these questions and their rationales appear on pages 157 to 159.

Case history questions

Lillian Bonner, age 24, was diagnosed with schizophrenia in her late teens. With treatment she usually is able to function with only very limited impairment, but currently is experiencing a second period of exacerbation.

1. To meet the *DSM-IV* diagnostic criteria for schizophrenia, how many of the characteristic symptoms (delusions, hallucinations, disorganized speech, grossly disorganized or catatonic behavior, negative symptoms) must Lillian have demonstrated?

    a. One or more
    b. Two or more
    c. Three or more
    d. Four or more

2. Currently Lillian displays disorganized speech. Which of the following is *not* descriptive of this criterion?
  a. Clang associations
  b. Echolalia
  c. Echopraxia
  d. Word salad

3. Lillian returned for treatment because, although she had wished her mother would die, she really didn't mean it and now wants the doctor to save her mother. This is a clear example of:
  a. an illusion.
  b. a delusion.
  c. ambivalence.
  d. magical thinking.

4. If Lillian were to develop hallucinations they would most likely be:
  a. auditory.
  b. olfactory.
  c. gustatory.
  d. tactile.

5. Given the widely accepted biochemical hypothesis for schizophrenia, drug therapy for Lillian will center on:
  a. neuroleptic drugs.
  b. antidepressants.
  c. anxiolytics.
  d. dopaminergics.

Additonal questions

6. Delusional disorders differ from schizophrenia in that they:
  a. are more apt to begin in early childhood.
  b. affect more men than women.
  c. affect more women than men.
  d. may be related to certain medical conditions.

7. Schizophrenic or delusional patients receiving clozapine require routine blood monitoring for:
  a. thrombocytopenia.
  b. aplastic anemia.
  c. agranulocytosis.
  d. hemolytic anemia.

CHAPTER 5

Mood Disorders

In these disorders, a person's mood becomes so intense and persistent that it interferes with his social and psychological function. Mood disorders include bipolar disorders and major depression.

Bipolar disorders

Marked by severe pathologic mood swings from hyperactivity and euphoria to sadness and depression, bipolar disorders involve various symptom combinations. Alternating episodes of mania and depression characterize type I bipolar disorder; recurrent depressive episodes and occasional manic episodes characterize type II.

In cyclothymia, a variant of bipolar disorder, numerous episodes of hypomania and depressive symptoms are too mild to meet the criteria for major depression or bipolar illness. (See *Cyclothymic disorder,* page 70.) In some patients, bipolar disorder assumes a seasonal pattern, marked by a cyclic relation between the onset of the mood episode and a particular 60-day period of the year.

The American Psychiatric Association estimates that 0.4% to 1.2% of adults experience bipolar disorder. This disorder is equally common among women and men, more common in higher socioeconomic groups, and associated with high levels of creativity. It can begin any time after adolescence, but first attacks usually occur between ages 20 and 35; about 35% of patients experience onset between ages 35 and 60. Before the onset of overt symptoms, many patients with bipolar disorder have an energetic and outgoing personality type with a history of wide mood swings.

Bipolar disorder recurs in 80% of patients; as they grow older, the attacks recur more frequently and last longer. This

Cyclothymic disorder

A chronic mood disturbance of at least 2 years' duration, cyclothymic disorder involves numerous episodes of hypomania or depressive symptoms that are not of sufficient severity or duration to qualify as a major depressive episode or a bipolar disorder.

Cyclothymia commonly starts in adolescence or early adulthood. Beginning insidiously, this disorder leads to persistent social and occupational dysfunction.

Signs and symptoms

In the hypomanic phase, the patient may experience insomnia; hyperactivity; inflated self-esteem; increased productivity and creativity; overinvolvement in pleasurable activities, including an in-creased sexual drive; physical restlessness; and rapid speech. Depressive symptoms may include insomnia, feelings of inadequacy, decreased productivity, social withdrawal, loss of libido, loss of interest in pleasurable activities, lethargy, depressed speech, and crying.

Diagnosis

A number of medical disorders (for example, endocrinopathies such as Cushing's disease, stroke, cerebrovascular accident, brain tumors, head trauma, and drug overdose) can produce a similar pattern of mood alteration. These organic causes must be ruled out before making a diagnosis of cyclothymic disorder.

---

illness is associated with a significant mortality; 20% of patients are victims of suicide, many just as the depression lifts.

Causes

The causes of bipolar disorders are unclear, but hereditary, biological, and psychological factors may play a part. For example, the incidence of bipolar disorder among relatives of affected patients is higher than in the general population and highest among maternal relatives. The closer the relationship, the greater the susceptibility. A child with one affected parent has a 25% chance of developing a bipolar disorder; a child with two affected parents, a 50% chance. The incidence of this illness in siblings is 20% to 25%; 66% to 96% in identical twins.

Although certain biochemical changes accompany mood swings, it's not clear whether these changes cause the mood swings or result from them. In both mania and depression, intracellular sodium concentration increases during illness and returns to normal with recovery.

Patients with mood disorders have a defect in the way the brain handles certain neurotransmitters – chemical messengers that shuttle nerve impulses between neurons. Low levels of dopamine and norepinephrine, for example, have been linked to depression, whereas excessively high levels of these chemicals are associated with mania.

Changes in the concentration of acetylcholine and serotonin also may play a role. Although neurobiologists have yet to prove that these chemical shifts cause bipolar disorders, it's widely assumed that most antidepressant medications work by modifying these neurotransmitter systems.

New data suggest that changes in the circadian rhythms that control hormone secretion, body temperature, and appetite may contribute to the development of a bipolar disorder.

Emotional or physical trauma, such as bereavement, disruption of an important relationship, or severe accidental injury, may precede the onset of bipolar disorder; however, bipolar disorder often appears without identifiable predisposing factors.

Manic episodes may follow a stressful event but are also associated with antidepressant therapy and childbirth. Major depressive episodes may be precipitated by chronic physical illness, psychoactive drug dependence, psychosocial stressors, and childbirth. Other familial influences, especially the early loss of a parent, parental depression, incest, or abuse, may predispose a person to depressive illness.

Signs and symptoms

Widely varying signs and symptoms depend on whether the patient is experiencing a manic or a depressive episode.

During the patient interview, the manic patient typically appears euphoric, expansive, or irritable, with little control over his activities and responses. He may describe hyperactive or excessive behavior, including elaborate plans for numerous social events, efforts to renew old acquaintances by telephoning friends at all hours of the night, buying sprees, or promiscuous sexual activity. He seldom hesitates to start projects for which he has little aptitude.

The patient's activities may have a bizarre quality, such as dressing in colorful or strange garments, wearing excessive makeup, or giving advice to passing strangers. He often expresses an inflated sense of self-esteem, ranging from uncritical self-confidence to marked grandiosity, which may be delusional.

Note the patient's speech patterns and concentration level. Accelerated speech, frequent changes of topic, and flight of ideas are common features of the manic phase. He's easily distracted and rapidly responds to external stimuli, such as background noise or a ringing telephone.

Physical examination of the manic patient may reveal signs of malnutrition and poor personal hygiene. He may report sleeping and eating less than usual.

Hypomania, more common than acute mania, can be recognized during the assessment interview by three classic symptoms: elated but unstable mood, pressured speech, and increased motor activity. The hypomanic patient may appear elated, hyperactive, easily distracted, talkative, irritable, impatient, impulsive, and full of energy, but seldom exhibits flight of ideas, delusions, or an absence of discretion and self-control.

The patient who experiences a depressive episode may report a loss of self-esteem, overwhelming inertia, social withdrawal, and feelings of hopelessness, apathy, or self-reproach. He may believe that he is wicked and deserves to be punished. His growing sadness, guilt, negativity, and fatigue place extraordinary burdens on his family.

During the history interview, the depressed patient may speak and respond slowly. He may complain of difficulty concentrating or thinking clearly but usually is not obviously disoriented or intellectually impaired.

Physical examination may reveal psychomotor retardation, lethargy, low muscle tonus, weight loss, slowed gait, and constipation. The patient also may report sleep disturbances (falling asleep, staying asleep, or early morning awakening), sexual dysfunction, headaches, chest pains, and a heaviness in the limbs. Typically, symptoms are worse in the morning and gradually subside as the day goes on.

His concerns about his health may become hypochondriacal: He may worry excessively about having cancer or some other severe illness. In an elderly patient, physical symptoms may be the only clues to depression.

Suicide is an ever-present risk, especially as the depression begins to lift. Then, a rising energy level may strengthen the patient's resolve to carry out suicidal plans.

The suicidal patient may also harbor homicidal ideas, thinking, for example, of killing his family either in anger or to spare them pain and disgrace.

Diagnosis

For characteristic findings in patients with this condition, see *Diagnosing bipolar disorders,* pages 74 to 76.

In addition, physical examination and laboratory tests, such as endocrine function studies, rule out medical causes of the mood disturbances, including intra-abdominal neoplasm, hypothyroidism, cardiac failure, cerebral arteriosclerosis, parkinsonism, psychoactive drug abuse, brain tumor, and uremia. Moreover, a review of the medications prescribed for other disorders may point to drug-induced depression or mania.

Treatment

Widely used to treat bipolar disorders, lithium proves highly effective in relieving and preventing manic episodes. The drug curbs the accelerated thought processes and hyperactive behavior without the sedating effect of antipsychotic drugs. In addition, it may prevent the recurrence of depressive episodes; however, it's ineffective in treating acute depression.

Lithium has a narrow therapeutic range, so treatment must be initiated cautiously and the dosage adjusted slowly. Therapeutic blood levels must be maintained for 7 to 10 days before effects appear; therefore, antipsychotic drugs often are used in the interim for sedation and symptomatic relief. Because lithium is excreted by the kidneys, any renal impairment necessitates withdrawal of the drug.

Anticonvulsants, such as carbamazepine, valproic acid, and clonazepam, are used to treat mood disorders either along with lithium or alone. For example, carbamazepine, a potent antimanic, often is effective in lithium-resistant patients.

Antidepressants are used to treat depressive symptoms, but they may trigger a manic episode.

Special considerations

Keep in mind the patient's physical and emotional needs.

For the manic patient

• Encourage the patient to eat.
• As the patient's symptoms subside, encourage him to assume responsibility for personal care.
• Provide emotional support, maintain a calm environment, and set realistic goals for behavior.

(Text continues on page 76.)

Diagnosing bipolar disorders

The diagnosis of a bipolar disorder is confirmed when the patient meets the criteria documented in the *DSM-IV.*

For a *manic episode:*
• A distinct period of abnormally and persistently elevated, expansive, or irritable mood lasting at least 1 week (or any duration if hospitalization is needed)
• During the mood disturbance period, at least three of the following symptoms must have persisted (four, if the mood is only irritable) and have been present to a significant degree. The symptoms are:
− inflated self-esteem or grandiosity
− decreased need for sleep
− unusual need to talk or pressure to keep talking
− flight of ideas or subjective experience that thoughts are racing
− distractibility
− increased level of goal-directed activity or psychomotor agitation
− excessive involvement in pleasurable activities that have a high potential for painful consequences.
• The symptoms do not meet the criteria for a mixed episode.
• The mood disturbance is sufficiently severe to cause one of the following to occur:
− marked impairment in occupational functioning or in usual social activities or relationships with others
− hospitalization to prevent harm to self or others
− evidence of psychotic features.
• The symptoms are not due to the direct physiologic effects of a substance or a general medical condition.

For a *hypomanic episode:*
• A distinct period of abnormally and persistently elevated, expansive, or irritable mood lasting at least 4 days that is clearly different from the usual nondepressed mood
• During the mood disturbance period, at least three of the following symptoms must have persisted (four, if the mood is only irritable) and have been present to a significant degree. The symptoms are:
− inflated self-esteem or grandiosity
− decreased need for sleep
− unusual need to talk or pressure to keep talking
− flight of ideas or subjective experience that thoughts are racing
− distractibility
− increased level of goal-directed activity or psychomotor agitation
− excessive involvement in pleasurable activities that have a high potential for painful consequences.
• The episode is associated with an unequivocal change in functioning that is uncharacteristic of the person when not symptomatic.
• Others can recognize the disturbance in mood and the change in functioning.
• The episode is not severe enough to markedly impair social or occupational functioning or to necessitate hospitalization to prevent harm to self or others, and no psychotic features are evident.
• The symptoms are not due to the direct physiologic effects of a substance or a general medical condition.

For a *bipolar I single manic episode:*
• Presence of only one manic episode and no past major depressive episodes
• The manic episode is not better accounted for by schizoaffective disorder and is not superimposed on schizophrenia, schizophreniform disorder, delusional disorder, or psychotic disorder not otherwise specified.

Diagnosing bipolar disorders *(continued)*

For a *bipolar I disorder, most recent episode hypomanic:*
• Currently (or most recently) in a hypomanic episode
• The person previously had at least one manic episode or mixed episode.
• The mood symptoms cause clinically significant distress or impairment in social, occupational, or other important areas of functioning.
• The first two exacerbations of the mood episode (above) are not better accounted for by schizoaffective disorder and are not superimposed on schizophrenia, schizophreniform disorder, delusional disorder, or psychotic disorder not otherwise specified.

For a *bipolar I disorder, most recent episode manic:*
• Currently (or most recently) in a manic episode
• The person previously had at least one major depressive episode, manic episode, or mixed episode.
• The first two exacerbations of mood episode (above) are not better accounted for by schizoaffective disorder and are not superimposed on schizophrenia, schizophreniform disorder, delusional disorder, or psychotic disorder not otherwise specified.

For a *bipolar I disorder, most recent episode mixed:*
• Currently (or most recently) in a mixed episode
• The person previously had at least one major depressive episode, manic episode, or mixed episode.
• The first two exacerbations of mood episode (above) are not better ac-

counted for by schizoaffective disorder and are not superimposed on schizophrenia, schizophreniform disorder, delusional disorder, or psychotic disorder not otherwise specified.

For a *bipolar I disorder, most recent episode depressed:*
• Currently (or most recently) in a major depressive episode
• The person previously had at least one manic episode or mixed episode.
• The first two exacerbations of mood episode above are not better accounted for by schizoaffective disorder and are not superimposed on schizophrenia, schizophreniform disorder, delusional disorder, or psychotic disorder not otherwise specified.

For a *bipolar I disorder, most recent episode unspecified:*
• Criteria, except for duration, are currently (or most recently) met for a manic, hypomanic, mixed, or major depressive episode.
• The person previously had at least one manic episode or mixed episode.
• The mood symptoms cause clinically significant distress or impairment in social, occupational, or other important areas of functioning.
• The first two exacerbations of mood episode (above) are not better accounted for by schizoaffective disorder and are not superimposed on schizophrenia, schizophreniform disorder, delusional disorder, or psychotic disorder not otherwise specified.
• The first two exacerbations of mood episode (above) are not due to the direct physiologic effects of a substance or a general medical condition.

(continued)

Diagnosing bipolar disorders (continued)

For a bipolar II disorder:
• Presence (or history) of one or more major depressive episodes
• Presence (or history) of at least one hypomanic episode
• The patient has never had a manic episode or a mixed episode.
• The first two exacerbations of mood episode (above) are not better ac-
counted for by schizoaffective disorder and are not superimposed on schizophrenia, schizophreniform disorder, delusional disorder, or psychotic disorder not otherwise specified.
• The symptoms cause clinically significant distress or impairment in social, occupational, or other important areas of functioning.

• Provide diversional activities suited to a short attention span; firmly discourage the patient if he tries to overextend himself.

• When necessary, reorient the patient to reality, and tactfully divert conversations when they become intimately involved with other patients or staff members.

• Set limits in a calm, clear, and self-confident manner for the manic patient's demanding, hyperactive, manipulative, and acting-out behaviors. Setting limits tells the patient you'll provide security and protection by refusing inappropriate and possibly harmful requests. Avoid leaving an opening for the patient to test or argue.

• Listen to requests attentively and with a neutral attitude, but avoid power struggles if a patient tries to put you on the spot for an immediate answer. Explain that you'll seriously consider the request and will respond later.

• Collaborate with other staff members to provide consistent responses to the patient's manipulations or acting out.

• Watch for early signs of frustration (when the patient's anger escalates from verbal threats to hitting an object). Tell the patient firmly that threats and hitting are unacceptable and that these behaviors show that he needs help to control his behavior. Then tell him that the staff will help him move to a quiet area and will help him control his behavior so he won't hurt himself or others. Staff members who have practiced as a team can work effectively to prevent acting-out behavior or to remove and confine a patient.

• Alert the staff team promptly when acting-out behavior escalates. It's safer to have help available before you need it than to try controlling an anxious or frightened patient by yourself.

• Once the incident is over and the patient is calm and in control, discuss his feelings with him and offer suggestions to prevent recurrence.

• If the patient is taking lithium, teach him and his family to discontinue the drug and notify the doctor if signs of toxicity, such as diarrhea, abdominal cramps, vomiting, unsteadiness, drowsiness, muscle weakness, polyuria, and tremors, occur.

For the depressed patient

• The depressed patient needs continual positive reinforcement to improve his self-esteem. Provide a structured routine, including activities to boost confidence and promote interaction with others (for instance, group therapy), and keep reassuring him that his depression will lift.

• Encourage the patient to talk or to write down his feelings if he's having trouble expressing them. Listen attentively and respectfully, and allow him time to formulate his thoughts if he seems sluggish. Record your observations and conversations.

• To prevent possible self-injury or suicide, remove harmful objects from the patient's environment (glass, belts, rope, bobby pins), observe him closely, and strictly supervise his medications. Institute suicide precautions as dictated by hospital policy.

• Don't forget the patient's physical needs. If he's too depressed to take care of himself, help him with personal hygiene. Encourage him to eat, or feed him, if necessary. If he's constipated, add high-fiber foods to his diet; offer small, frequent meals; and encourage physical activity. To help him sleep, give back rubs or warm milk at bedtime.

• If the patient is taking an antidepressant, watch for signs of mania.

Major depression

Also known as unipolar disorder, major depression is a syndrome of a persistently sad, dysphoric mood accompanied by disturbances in sleep and appetite, lethargy, and an inability to experience pleasure (anhedonia). Major depression occurs in up to 17% of adults, affecting all racial, ethnic, and socioeconomic groups. It affects both sexes but is more common in women.

About half of all depressed patients experience a single episode and recover completely; the rest have at least one recurrence. Major depression can profoundly alter social, family, and occupational functioning. However, suicide is the most serious complication of major depression, resulting when the patient's feelings of worthlessness, guilt, and hopelessness are so overwhelming that he no longer considers life worth living. Nearly twice as many women as men attempt suicide, but men are far more likely to succeed. (See *Suicide prevention guidelines.*)

Causes

The multiple causes of depression are not completely understood. Current research suggests possible genetic, familial, biochemical, physical, psychological, and social causes. Psychological causes (the focus of many medical interventions) may include feelings of helplessness and vulnerability, anger, hopelessness and pessimism, and low self-esteem; they may be related to abnormal character and behavior patterns and troubled personal relations. In many patients, the history identifies a specific personal loss or severe stress that probably interacts with a person's predisposition to provoke major depression.

Depression may be secondary to a specific medical condition, for example, metabolic disturbances, such as hypoxia and hypercalcemia; endocrine disorders, such as diabetes and Cushing's disease; neurologic diseases, such as Parkinson's and Alzheimer's disease; cancer (especially of the pancreas); viral and bacterial infections, such as influenza and pneumonia; cardiovascular disorders such as congestive heart failure; pulmonary disorders such as chronic obstructive lung disease; musculoskeletal disorders such as

Suicide prevention guidelines

When your patient has a diagnosis of major depression, keep in mind the following guidelines.

Assess for clues to suicide
Be alert for the patient's suicidal thoughts, threats, and messages; hoarding medication; talking about death and feelings of futility; giving away prized possessions; describing a suicide plan; and changing his behavior, especially as the depression begins to lift.

Provide a safe environment
Check patient areas and correct dangerous conditions, such as exposed pipes, windows without safety glass, and access to the roof or open balconies.

Remove dangerous objects
Take away such objects as belts, razors, suspenders, light cords, glass, knives, nail files and clippers, and metal and hard plastic objects.

Consult with staff
Recognize and document both verbal and nonverbal suicidal behaviors; keep others informed; share data with all staff; clarify the patient's specific restrictions; assess risk and plan for observation; clarify day and night staff responsibilities and frequency of consultation.

Observe the suicidal patient
Be alert when the patient is using a sharp object (to prevent injury such as while shaving), taking medication, or using the bathroom (to prevent hanging or other injury). Assign the patient to a room near the nurses' station and with another patient. Continuously observe the acutely suicidal patient.

Maintain personal contact
Help the suicidal patient feel that he's not alone or without resources or hope. Encourage continuity of care and consistency of primary nurses. Building emotional ties to others is the ultimate technique for preventing suicide.

degenerative arthritis; GI disorders such as irritable bowel syndrome; genitourinary problems such as incontinence; collagen vascular diseases such as lupus; and anemias.

Drugs prescribed for medical and psychiatric conditions, as well as many commonly abused substances, can also cause depression. Examples include antihypertensives, psychotropics, antiparkinsonian drugs, narcotic and nonnarcotic analgesics, numerous cardiovascular medications, oral antidiabetics, antimicrobials, corticosteroids, chemotherapeutic agents, cimetidine, and alcohol.

Signs and symptoms

The primary features of major depression are a predominantly sad mood and a loss of interest or pleasure in daily activities. The patient may complain of feeling "down in the

Dysthymic disorder: A chronic affective disorder

This disorder is characterized by a chronic dysphoric mood (irritable mood in children), persisting at least 2 years in adults and 1 year in children and adolescents.

Signs and symptoms
During periods of depression, the patient also may experience poor appetite or overeating, insomnia or hypersomnia, low energy or fatigue, low self-esteem, poor concentration or difficulty making decisions, and feelings of hopelessness.

Diagnosis
Dysthymic disorder is confirmed when the patient exhibits at least two of the symptoms named above nearly every day, with intervening normal moods lasting no more than 2 months during a 2-year period.

Dysthymic disorder typically begins in childhood, adolescence, or early adulthood and causes only mild social or occupational impairment. In adults, it's more common in women; in children and adolescents, it's equally common in both sexes.

---

dumps," express doubts about his self-worth or ability to cope, or simply appear unhappy and apathetic. He also may report feeling angry or anxious. Other common signs include difficulty concentrating or thinking clearly, distractibility, and indecisiveness. Take special note if the patient reveals suicidal thoughts, a preoccupation with death, or previous suicide attempts.

The psychosocial history may reveal life problems or losses that can account for the depression. Alternatively, the patient's medical history may implicate a physical disorder or the use of prescription, nonprescription, or illegal drugs that can cause depression.

The patient may report an increase or decrease in appetite, sleep disturbances (for example, insomnia or early awakening), a lack of interest in sexual activity, constipation, or diarrhea. Other signs you may note during a physical examination include agitation (such as hand wringing or restlessness) and psychomotor retardation (for example, slowed speech). (To distinguish major depression from dysthymia, a disorder with similar symptoms, see *Dysthymic disorder: A chronic affective disorder.*)

Diagnosis

For characteristic findings in patients with this condition, see *Diagnosing major depression.*

Diagnosing major depression

A patient is diagnosed with major depression when he fulfills the following criteria for a single major depressive episode put forth in the *DSM-IV:*

• At least five of the following symptoms must have been present during the same 2-week period and must represent a change from previous functioning; one of these symptoms must be either depressed mood or loss of interest in previously pleasurable activities:

−depressed mood (irritable mood in children and adolescents) most of the day, nearly every day, as indicated by either a subjective account or observation by others

−markedly diminished interest or pleasure in all, or almost all, activities most of the day, nearly every day

−significant weight loss or weight gain when not dieting or decrease or increase in appetite nearly every day (in children, consider failure to make expected weight gains)

−insomnia or hypersomnia nearly every day

−psychomotor agitation or retardation nearly every day

−fatigue or loss of energy nearly every day

−feelings of worthlessness or excessive or inappropriate guilt nearly every day

−diminished ability to think or concentrate, or indecisiveness, nearly every day

−recurrent thoughts of death, recurrent suicidal ideation without a specific plan, a suicide attempt, or a specific plan for committing suicide.

• The symptoms do not meet criteria for a mixed episode.

• The symptoms cause clinically significant distress or impairment in social, occupational, or other important areas of functioning.

• The symptoms are not due to the direct physiologic effects of a substance or a general medical condition.

• The symptoms are not better accounted for by bereavement, persist for longer than 2 months, or are characterized by marked functional impairment, morbid preoccupation with worthlessness, suicidal ideation, psychotic symptoms, or psychomotor retardation.

The findings of major depression are supported by psychological tests, such as the Beck Depression Inventory, which may help determine the onset, severity, duration, and progression of depressive symptoms. Toxicology screening may suggest a drug-induced depression.

Treatment Depression is difficult to treat, especially in children, adolescents, elderly patients, and those with a history of chronic disease. The primary treatment methods are drug therapy, electroconvulsive therapy (ECT), and psychotherapy.

Drug therapy includes tricyclic antidepressants (such as amitriptyline), monoamine oxidase (MAO) inhibitors (for example, isocarboxazid), maprotiline, trazodone, bupropion, and serotonin reuptake inhibitors (such as fluoxetine).

Tricyclic antidepressants (TCAs), the most widely used of the antidepressant drugs, prevent the reuptake of norepinephrine or serotonin or both into the presynaptic nerve endings, resulting in increased synaptic concentrations of these neurotransmitters. They also cause a gradual loss in the number of beta-adrenergic receptors.

Selective serotonin reuptake inhibitors (SSRIs), including fluoxetine, paroxetine, and sertraline, are increasingly the drugs of choice. They are effective and produce fewer adverse effects — although they are associated with sleep and GI problems and alterations in sexual desire and function.

MAO inhibitors block the enzymatic degradation of norepinephrine and serotonin. These agents often are prescribed for patients with atypical depression (for example, depression marked by an increase in appetite and the need for sleep, rather than anorexia and insomnia) and for some patients who fail to respond to the TCAs. The MAO inhibitors are associated with a high risk of toxicity; patients treated with one of these drugs must be able to comply with the necessary dietary restrictions. Conservative doses of an MAO inhibitor may be combined with a TCA for patients refractory to either drug alone.

Maprotiline is a potent blocker of norepinephrine uptake, whereas trazodone is a selective serotonin uptake blocker. The mechanism of action of bupropion is unknown.

When a depressed patient is incapacitated, actively suicidal, or psychotically depressed, or when antidepressants are contraindicated or ineffective, ECT often is the treatment of choice. Six to 12 treatments usually are required, although improvement often is evident after only a few treatments. Researchers hypothesize that the treatment affects the same receptor sites as antidepressant medications.

Short-term psychotherapy also is effective in the treatment of major depression. Many psychiatrists believe that the best results are achieved with a combination of individual, family, or group psychotherapy and medication. After resolution of the acute episode, patients with a history of recurrent depression may be maintained on low doses of antidepressant drugs as a preventive measure.

Special considerations

• Share your observations of the patient's behavior with him. For instance, you might say, "You're sitting all by yourself, looking very sad. Is that how you feel?" Because the patient may think and react sluggishly, speak slowly and allow ample time for him to respond. Avoid feigned cheerfulness. However, don't hesitate to laugh with the patient and point out the value of humor.

• Encourage the patient to talk about and write down his feelings. Show him he's important by listening attentively and respectfully, preventing interruptions, and avoiding judgmental responses.

• Provide a structured routine, including noncompetitive activities, to build the patient's self-confidence and encourage interaction with others. Urge him to join group activities and to socialize.

• Reassure the patient that he can help ease his depression by expressing his feelings, participating in pleasurable activities, and improving grooming and hygiene.

• Ask the patient if he thinks of death or suicide. Such thoughts signal an immediate need for consultation and assessment. Failure to detect suicidal thoughts early may encourage the patient to attempt suicide. The risk of suicide increases as the depression lifts.

• While caring for the patient's psychological needs, don't forget his physical needs. If he's too depressed to take care of himself, help him with personal hygiene. Encourage him to eat, or feed him, if necessary. If he's constipated, add high-fiber foods to his diet; offer small, frequent feedings; and encourage physical activity and fluid intake. Offer warm milk or back rubs at bedtime to improve sleep.

• If the patient has been prescribed an antidepressant, monitor for evidence of seizures. Some antidepressants significantly lower the seizure threshold.

• Recognize that it may take several weeks for the antidepressants to produce an effect.

• Teach the patient about his depression. Emphasize that effective methods are available to relieve his symptoms. Help him to recognize distorted perceptions and link them to his depression. Once the patient learns to recognize depressive thought patterns, he can consciously begin to substitute self-affirming thoughts.

• Instruct the patient about prescribed medications. Stress the need for compliance and review adverse reactions. For drugs that produce strong anticholinergic effects, such as amitriptyline and amoxapine, suggest sugarless gum or hard candy to relieve dry mouth. Many antidepressants are sedating (for example, amitriptyline and trazodone); warn the patient to avoid activities that require alertness, including driving and operating mechanical equipment.

• Caution the patient taking a TCA to avoid drinking alcoholic beverages or taking other central nervous system depressants during therapy.

• If the patient is taking an MAO inhibitor, emphasize that he must avoid foods that contain tyramine, caffeine, or tryptophan. Emphasize that the ingestion of tyramine can cause a hypertensive crisis. Examples of foods that contain these substances are cheese; sour cream; beer, chianti, or sherry; pickled herring; liver; canned figs; raisins; bananas; avocados; chocolate; soy sauce; fava beans; yeast extracts; meat tenderizers; coffee; and colas.

Self-test questions

You can quickly review your comprehension of this chapter on mood disorders by answering the following questions. The correct answers to these questions and their rationales appear on pages 159 and 160.

1. Bipolar II disorder differs from bipolar I disorder in that in bipolar II disorder there has (have) never been:
    a. major depressive episodes.
    b. hypomanic episodes.
    c. a manic episode.
    d. significant functional impairment.

2. Cyclothymic disorder is defined by:

a. a seasonal pattern characterized by a cyclic relationship between the mood episode onset and a particular season of the year.
b. numerous episodes of hypomania and depressive symptoms too mild to meet the criteria for bipolar illnesses or major depression.
c. episodes of mixed mania and depression.
d. mood episodes that may be related to a schizoaffective disorder.

3. To relieve and prevent manic episodes and perhaps prevent depressive episodes in bipolar I disorder, the patient is most apt to be prescribed:
a. carbamazepine.
b. lithium.
c. clonazepam.
d. valproic acid.

Case history questions

Janet Mimms, age 33, married and the mother of four young children, has experienced multiple episodes of depression that seem to be increasingly frequent.

4. The most serious complication of major depression is:
a. altered social and family functioning.
b. a feeling of worthlessness.
c. a feeling of hopelessness.
d. suicide.

5. While depression can result from a medical condition or prescribed or abused drugs, these have been ruled out in Janet's case. Suspicion would now turn to:
a. genetic and familial causes.
b. societal causes.
c. biochemical causes.
d. multiple causes.

6. Janet demonstrates many of the criteria for the *DSM-IV* depression classification nearly every day. One of these criteria must be a depressed mood or:
a. insomnia or hypersomnia.
b. feelings of worthlessness or excessive or inappropriate guilt.

    c. loss of interest in previously pleasurable activities.
    d. diminished ability to think, concentrate, or make decisions.

7. Janet receives fluoxetine, a selective serotonin reuptake inhibitor. These drugs are increasingly chosen to treat depression because they:
    a. prevent recurrence.
    b. have fewer disturbing adverse effects.
    c. require only minimal dietary modifications.
    d. work well for patients who fail to respond to tricyclic antidepressants.

8. If Janet relapses, her psychiatrist plans to use ECT. How many treatments are usually required?
    a. 1 to 2
    b. 2 to 4
    c. 4 to 8
    d. 6 to 12

CHAPTER 6

Anxiety Disorders

A component of most psychological disorders and many organic disorders, anxiety is a common complaint of most hospitalized patients. Diagnosed anxiety disorders are classified into five basic types: phobias, generalized anxiety disorder, panic disorder, obsessive-compulsive disorder, and posttraumatic stress disorder.

Phobias

Defined as a persistent and irrational fear of a specific object, activity, or situation, a phobia results in a compelling desire to avoid the perceived hazard. The patient recognizes that his fear is out of proportion to any actual danger, but he can't control it or explain it away. Three types of phobias exist: agoraphobia, the fear of being alone or of open space; social phobia, the fear of embarrassing oneself in public; and specific phobia, the fear of a single, specific object, such as animals or heights.

Seven percent of all Americans suffer from a phobic disorder. In fact, phobias are the most common psychiatric disorders in women and the second most common in men. More men than women experience social phobias, whereas agoraphobia and specific phobias are more common in women. The onset of a social phobia typically is in late childhood or early adolescence; a specific phobia usually begins in childhood. Most phobic patients have no family history of psychiatric illness, including phobias.

Both agoraphobia and social phobia tend to be chronic, but new treatments are improving the prognosis. A specific phobia usually resolves spontaneously as the child matures.

Causes

A phobia develops when anxiety about an object or a situation compels the patient to avoid it.

The precise cause of most phobias is unknown. Psychoanalytic theory holds that the phobia is actually repression and displacement of an internal conflict. Behavioral theorists view phobia as a stimulus-response reflex, in which the patient avoids a situation or object that causes anxiety.

Signs and symptoms

The phobic patient typically reports signs of severe anxiety when confronted with the feared object or situation. A patient with agoraphobia, for example, may complain of dizziness, a sensation of falling, depersonalization or a feeling of unreality, loss of bladder or bowel control, vomiting, or cardiac distress when he leaves home or crosses a bridge. Similarly, a patient who fears flying may report that he begins to sweat, his heart pounds, and he feels panicky and short of breath when he's on an airplane.

A patient who routinely avoids the object of his phobia may report a loss of self-esteem and feelings of weakness, cowardice, or ineffectiveness. If he hasn't mastered the phobia, he also may exhibit signs of mild depression.

Diagnosis

For characteristic findings in patients with this condition, see *Diagnosing phobias.*

Treatment

The effectiveness of treatment depends on the severity of the patient's phobia. Because phobic behavior may never be completely cured, the goal of treatment is to help the patient function effectively.

Antianxiety and antidepressant drugs may help relieve symptoms in patients with agoraphobia.

Systematic desensitization, a behavioral therapy, may be more effective than drugs, especially if it includes encouragement, instruction, and suggestion.

In some cities, phobia clinics and group therapy are available. People who have recovered from phobias can often help other phobic patients.

Special considerations

• Provide for the patient's safety and comfort and monitor fluid and food intake as needed. Certain phobias may inhibit food or fluid intake, disturb hygiene, and disrupt the patient's ability to rest.

Diagnosing phobias

The diagnosis of all three types of phobias is based on criteria put forth in the *DSM-IV.*

Agoraphobia

Fear of being in places or situations from which escape might be difficult or embarrassing or in which help might be unavailable if an unexpected or situationally predisposed panic attack or paniclike symptoms occur. Agoraphobic fears typically involve characteristic clusters of situations that include being outside the home alone, being in a crowd or standing in a line, being on a bridge, and traveling in a bus, train, or automobile.
• The situations are avoided or otherwise endured with marked distress or with anxiety about having a panic attack or paniclike symptoms, or they require the presence of a companion.
• The anxiety or phobic avoidance is not better accounted for by another mental disorder, such as social phobia, specific phobia, obsessive-compulsive disorder, posttraumatic stress disorder, or separation anxiety disorder.

Social phobia

A persistent fear of one or more social or performance situations in which the person is exposed to unfamiliar people or possible scrutiny by others. The person fears that he may act in a way that will be humiliating or embarrassing.
• Exposure to the feared social situation almost invariably provokes anxiety, which may take the form of a situationally bound or situationally predisposed panic attack.
• The person recognizes that the fear is excessive or unreasonable.

• The feared social or performance situations are avoided or endured with intense anxiety or distress.
• The avoidance, anxious anticipation, or distress in the feared social or performance situation interferes with the person's normal routine, occupational functioning, or social activities or relationships, or there is marked distress about having the phobia.
• In individuals under age 18, the duration is at least 6 months.
• The fear or avoidance is not due to the direct physiologic effects of a substance or a general medical condition and is not better accounted for by another mental disorder.
• If the person has a general medical condition or another mental disorder, the person's social fear is unrelated to the medical or mental conditions.

Specific phobia

Marked and persistent fear that is excessive or unreasonable and cued by the presence or anticipation of a specific object or situation.
• Exposure to the phobic stimulus almost invariably provokes an immediate anxiety response, which may take the form of a situationally bound or situationally predisposed panic attack.
• The person recognizes that the fear is excessive or unreasonable.
• The person avoids the situation or endures it with intense anxiety or distress.
• The avoidance, anxious anticipation, or distress in the feared situation significantly interferes with the person's normal routine, occupational functioning, or social activities or relationships, or there is marked distress about having the phobia.

(continued)

Diagnosing phobias *(continued)*

• In individuals under age 18, the duration is at least 6 months.
• The anxiety, panic attacks, or phobic avoidance associated with the specific object or situation are not better accounted for by another mental disorder, such as obsessive-compulsive disorder, posttraumatic stress disorder, separation anxiety disorder, social phobia, panic disorder with agoraphobia, or agoraphobia without history of panic disorder.

• No matter how illogical the patient's phobia seems, avoid the urge to trivialize his fears. Remember that this behavior represents an essential coping mechanism.
• Ask the patient how he normally copes with the fear. When he's able to face the fear, encourage him to verbalize and explore his personal strengths and resources with you.
• Don't let the patient withdraw completely. If he's being treated as an outpatient, suggest small steps to overcome his fears such as planning a brief shopping trip with a supportive family member or friend.
• In social phobias, the patient fears criticism. Encourage him to interact with others and provide continuous support and positive reinforcement.
• Support participation in psychotherapy, including desensitization therapy. However, don't force insight. Challenging the patient may aggravate his anxiety or lead to panic attacks.
• Teach the patient specific relaxation techniques, such as listening to music and meditating.
• Suggest ways to channel the patient's energy and relieve stress (such as running and creative activities).

Generalized anxiety disorder

Anxiety is a feeling of apprehension that some describe as an exaggerated feeling of impending doom, dread, or uneasiness. Unlike fear—a reaction to danger from a specific external source—anxiety is a reaction to an internal threat, such as an unacceptable impulse or a repressed thought that's straining to reach a conscious level.

A rational response to a real threat, occasional anxiety is a normal part of life. Overwhelming anxiety, however, can result in generalized anxiety disorder—uncontrollable, unreasonable worry that persists for at least 6 months and narrows perceptions or interferes with normal functioning. Recent evidence shows that the prevalence of generalized anxiety disorder is greater than previously thought and may be even greater than that of depression.

Causes

Theorists share a common premise: Conflict, whether intrapsychic, sociopersonal, or interpersonal, promotes an anxiety state.

Signs and symptoms

Generalized anxiety disorder can begin at any age but typically has an onset in one's 20s and 30s. It is equally common in men and women. Psychological or physiologic symptoms of anxious states vary with the degree of anxiety. Mild anxiety mainly causes psychological symptoms, with unusual self-awareness and alertness to the environment. Moderate anxiety leads to selective inattention, yet with the ability to concentrate on a single task. Severe anxiety causes an inability to concentrate on more than scattered details of a task. A panic state with acute anxiety causes a complete loss of concentration, often with unintelligible speech.

Physical examination of the patient with generalized anxiety disorder may reveal symptoms of motor tension, including trembling, muscle aches and spasms, headaches, and an inability to relax. Autonomic signs and symptoms include shortness of breath, tachycardia, sweating, and abdominal complaints.

In addition, the patient may startle easily and complain of feeling apprehensive, fearful, or angry and of having difficulty concentrating, eating, and sleeping. The medical, psychiatric, and psychosocial histories fail to identify a specific physical or environmental cause of the anxiety.

Diagnosis

For characteristic findings in patients with this condition, see *Diagnosing generalized anxiety disorder,* page 92.

In addition, laboratory tests must exclude organic causes of the patient's signs and symptoms, such as hyperthyroid-

Diagnosing generalized anxiety disorder

When the patient's symptoms match criteria documented in the *DSM-IV*, the diagnosis of generalized anxiety disorder is confirmed. The criteria include the following:

• The excessive anxiety and worry about a number of events or activities occur more days than not for at least 6 months.

• The person finds it difficult to control the worry.

• The anxiety and worry are associated with at least three of the following six symptoms:
— restlessness or feeling keyed up or on edge
— being easily fatigued
— difficulty concentrating or mind going blank
— irritability
— muscle tension
— sleep disturbance (difficulty falling or staying asleep, or restless, unsatisfying sleep).

• The focus of the anxiety and worry is not confined to features of an Axis I disorder.

• The anxiety, worry, or physical symptoms cause clinically significant distress or impairment in social, occupational, or other important areas of functioning.

• The disturbance is not due to the direct physiologic effects of a substance or a general medical condition and does not occur exclusively during a mood disorder, a psychotic disorder, or a pervasive developmental disorder.

---

ism, pheochromocytoma, coronary artery disease, supraventricular tachycardia, and Ménière's disease. For example, an electrocardiogram can rule out myocardial ischemia in a patient who complains of chest pain. Blood tests, including complete blood count, white blood cell differential, and serum lactate and calcium levels, can rule out hypocalcemia.

Because anxiety is the central feature of other mental disorders, psychiatric evaluation must rule out phobias, obsessive-compulsive disorders, depression, and acute schizophrenia.

Treatment

A combination of drug therapy and psychotherapy may help a patient with generalized anxiety disorder. The benzodiazepine antianxiety drugs may relieve mild anxiety and improve the patient's ability to cope. Tricyclic antidepressants or higher doses of benzodiazepines may relieve severe anxiety and panic attacks. Buspirone, an antianxiety drug, causes less sedation and less risk of physical and psychological dependence than the benzodiazepines.

Psychotherapy for generalized anxiety disorder has two goals: helping the patient identify and deal with the cause of the anxiety and eliminating environmental factors that precipitate an anxious reaction. In addition, the patient can learn relaxation techniques, such as deep breathing, progressive muscle relaxation, focused relaxation, and visualization.

Special considerations

• Stay with the patient when he's anxious, and encourage him to discuss his feelings. Reduce environmental stimuli and remain calm.

• Administer antianxiety drugs or tricyclic antidepressants as necessary, and evaluate the patient's response. Teach the patient about prescribed medications, including the need for compliance with the medication regimen. Review adverse reactions.

• Teach the patient effective coping strategies and relaxation techniques. Help him identify stressful situations that trigger his anxiety, and provide positive reinforcement when he uses alternative coping strategies.

Panic disorder

Characterized by recurrent episodes of intense apprehension, terror, and impending doom, panic disorder represents anxiety in its most severe form. Initially unpredictable, these "panic attacks" may come to be associated with specific situations or tasks. The disorder often exists concurrently with agoraphobia. Equal numbers of men and women are affected by panic disorder alone, whereas panic disorder with agoraphobia occurs about twice as often in women.

Panic disorder typically has an onset in late adolescence or early adulthood, often in response to a sudden loss. It also may be triggered by severe separation anxiety experienced during early childhood. Without treatment, panic disorder can persist for years, with alternating exacerbations and remissions. The patient with panic disorder is at high risk for a psychoactive substance abuse disorder, resorting to alcohol or anxiolytics in an attempt to relieve his fear.

Causes

Like other anxiety disorders, panic disorder may stem from a combination of physical and psychological factors. For example, some theorists emphasize the role of stressful events or unconscious conflicts that occur early in childhood.

Recent evidence indicates that alterations in brain biochemistry, especially in norepinephrine, serotonin, and gamma-aminobutyric acid activity, may also contribute to panic disorder.

Signs and symptoms

The patient with panic disorder typically complains of repeated episodes of unexpected apprehension, fear or, rarely, intense discomfort. These panic attacks may last for minutes or hours and leave the patient shaken, fearful, and exhausted. They occur several times a week, sometimes even daily. Because the attacks occur spontaneously, without exposure to a known anxiety-producing situation, the patient often worries between attacks about when the next episode will occur.

Physical examination of the patient during a panic attack may reveal signs of intense anxiety, such as hyperventilation, tachycardia, trembling, and profuse sweating. He may also complain of difficulty breathing, digestive disturbances, and chest pain.

Diagnosis

For characteristic findings in patients with this condition, see *Diagnosing panic disorder.*

Because many medical conditions can mimic panic disorder, additional tests may be ordered to rule out an organic basis for the symptoms. For example, tests for serum glucose levels rule out hypoglycemia, studies of urine catecholamines and vanillylmandelic acid rule out pheochromocytoma, and thyroid function tests rule out hyperthyroidism.

Urine and serum toxicology tests reveal the presence of psychoactive substances that can precipitate panic attacks, including barbiturates, caffeine, and amphetamines.

Treatment

Panic disorder may respond to behavioral therapy, supportive psychotherapy, or drug therapy, singly or in combination. Behavioral therapy works best when agoraphobia accompanies panic disorder because the identification of anxiety-inducing situations is easier.

Diagnosing panic disorder

The diagnosis of panic disorder is confirmed when the patient meets the criteria put forth in the *DSM-IV.*

Panic attack
A discrete period of intense fear or discomfort in which at least four of the following symptoms develop abruptly and reach a peak within 10 minutes:
• palpitations, pounding heart, or tachycardia
• sweating
• trembling or shaking
• shortness of breath or smothering sensations
• feeling of choking
• chest pain or discomfort
• nausea or abdominal distress
• dizziness or faintness
• depersonalization or derealization
• fear of losing control or going crazy
• fear of dying
• numbness or tingling sensations (paresthesia)
• hot flashes or chills.

Panic disorder without agoraphobia
• The person experiences recurrent unexpected panic attacks and at least one of the attacks has been followed by 1 month (or more) or one (or more) of the following:
—persistent concern about having additional attacks
—worry about the implications of the attack or its consequences

—a significant change in behavior related to the attacks.
• The panic attacks are not due to the direct physiologic effects of a substance or a general medical condition.
• The panic attacks are not better accounted for by another mental disorder, such as social phobia, specific phobia, obsessive-compulsive disorder, posttraumatic stress disorder, or separation anxiety disorder.

Panic disorder with agoraphobia
• The person experiences recurrent unexpected panic attacks and at least one of the attacks has been followed by 1 month (or more) or one (or more) of the following:
—persistent concern about having additional attacks
—worry about the implications of the attack or its consequences
—a significant change in behavior related to the attacks.
• The person exhibits agoraphobia.
• The panic attacks are not due to the direct physiologic effects of a substance or a general medical condition.
• The panic attacks are not better accounted for by another mental disorder, such as social phobia, specific phobia, obsessive-compulsive disorder, posttraumatic stress disorder, or separation anxiety disorder.

Psychotherapy commonly uses cognitive techniques to enable the patient to view anxiety-provoking situations more realistically and to recognize panic symptoms as a misinterpretation of essentially harmless physical sensations.

Drug therapy includes antianxiety drugs, such as diazepam, alprazolam, and clonazepam, and beta blockers such as propranolol to provide symptomatic relief. Antidepressants, including tricyclic antidepressants, selective serotonin reuptake inhibitors, and monoamine oxidase inhibitors, are also effective.

Special considerations

• Stay with the patient until the attack subsides. If left alone, he may become even more anxious.

• Maintain a calm, serene approach. Use statements such as "I won't let anything here hurt you" and "I'll stay with you" to assure the patient that you're in control of the immediate situation. Avoid insincere expressions of reassurance.

• The patient's perceptual field may be narrowed, and excessive stimuli may cause him to feel overwhelmed. Dim bright lights or raise dim lights as necessary. If the patient loses control, remove him to a smaller, quieter space.

• The patient may be so overwhelmed that he cannot follow lengthy or complicated processes. Speak in short, simple sentences, and slowly give one direction at a time. Avoid giving lengthy explanations and asking too many questions.

• Allow the patient to pace around the room (provided he isn't belligerent) to help expend energy. Show him how to take slow, deep breaths if he's hyperventilating.

• Avoid touching the patient until you've established rapport. Unless he trusts you, he may be too stimulated or frightened to find touch reassuring.

• Administer medication as necessary.

• During and after a panic attack, encourage the patient to express his feelings. Discuss his fears and help him identify situations or events that trigger the attacks.

• Teach the patient relaxation techniques. Point out ways he can use these methods to relieve stress or avoid a panic attack.

• Review with the patient any adverse effects of the drugs he'll be taking. Caution him that abrupt withdrawal from a drug could cause severe symptoms.

• Encourage the patient and the family to use community resources such as the Anxiety Disorders Association of America.

Obsessive-compulsive disorder

Obsessive thoughts and compulsive behaviors represent recurring efforts to control overwhelming anxiety, guilt, or unacceptable impulses that persistently enter the consciousness.

The word "obsession" refers to a recurrent idea, thought, impulse, or image that is intrusive and inappropriate and causes marked anxiety or distress. A compulsion is a ritualistic, repetitive, and involuntary defensive behavior. Performing a compulsive behavior reduces the patient's anxiety and reinforces the probability that the behavior will recur. Compulsions are often associated with obsessions.

Patients with obsessive-compulsive disorder are prone to abuse psychoactive substances, such as alcohol and anxiolytics, in an attempt to relieve their anxiety. In addition, major depression and other anxiety disorders often coexist with obsessive-compulsive states.

Mild forms of the disorder are relatively common in the population at large. Generally, an obsessive-compulsive disorder is chronic, often with remissions and flare-ups.

Causes

The cause of obsessive-compulsive disorder is unknown. Some studies suggest the possibility of brain lesions, but the most useful research and clinical studies base an explanation on psychological theories. In addition, major depression, organic brain syndrome, and schizophrenia may contribute to the onset of obsessive-compulsive disorder.

Signs and symptoms

The psychiatric history of a patient with this disorder may reveal the presence of obsessive thoughts, words, or mental images that persistently and involuntarily invade the consciousness. Some common obsessions include thoughts of violence (such as stabbing, shooting, maiming, or hitting), thoughts of contamination (images of dirt, germs, or feces), repetitive doubts and worry about a tragic event, and repeating or counting images, words, or objects in the environment. The patient recognizes that the obsessions are a product of his own mind and that they interfere with normal daily activities.

The patient's history also may reveal the presence of compulsions, irrational and recurring impulses to repeat a certain behavior. Common compulsions include repetitive touching, sometimes combined with counting; doing and undoing (opening and closing doors, rearranging things); washing (especially hands); and checking (to be sure no tragedy has occurred). The patient's anxiety often is so strong that he will avoid the situation or the object that evokes the impulse.

When the obsessive-compulsive phenomena are mental, observation may reveal no behavioral abnormalities. However, compulsive acts may be observed, although feelings of shame, nervousness, or embarrassment may prompt the patient to try limiting these acts to his own private time.

Also evaluate the impact of obsessive-compulsive phenomena on the patient's normal routine. He'll typically report moderate to severe impairment of social and occupational functioning.

Diagnosis

For characteristic findings in patients with this condition, see *Diagnosing obsessive-compulsive disorder.*

Treatment

Obsessive-compulsive disorder is tenacious, but with treatment, improvement occurs in 60% to 70% of patients. Current treatment usually involves a combination of medication and cognitive behavioral therapy. Other psychotherapies may also be helpful.

Effective medications include clomipramine, a tricyclic antidepressant; selective serotonin reuptake inhibitors, such as fluoxetine, paroxetine, sertraline, and fluvoxamine; and the benzodiazepine clonazepam.

Behavioral therapies — aversion therapy, thought stopping, thought switching, flooding, implosion therapy, and response prevention — have also been effective (see *Behavioral therapies,* page 100).

Special considerations

• Approach the patient unhurriedly.
• Provide an accepting atmosphere; don't show shock, amusement, or criticism of the ritualistic behavior.
• Keep the patient's physical health in mind. For example, compulsive hand washing may cause skin breakdown, and rituals or preoccupations may cause inadequate food and

Diagnosing obsessive-compulsive disorder

The diagnosis of obsessive-compulsive disorder is made when the patient's signs and symptoms meet the established criteria put forth in the *DSM-IV.*

Either obsessions or compulsions
Obsessions are defined by all of the following:
• Recurrent and persistent thoughts, impulses, or images that are experienced, at some time during the disturbance, as intrusive and inappropriate and that cause marked anxiety or distress.
• The thoughts, impulses, or images are not simply excessive worries about real-life problems.
• The person attempts to ignore or suppress such thoughts or impulses or to neutralize them with some other thought or action.
• The person recognizes that the obsessions are the products of his mind and not externally imposed.

Compulsions are defined by all of the following:
• Repetitive behaviors or mental acts performed by the person who feels driven to perform in response to an obsession or according to rules that must be applied rigidly.
• The behavior or mental acts are aimed at preventing or reducing distress or preventing some dreaded event or situa-

tion. However, either the activity is not connected in a realistic way with what it is designed to neutralize or prevent, or it is clearly excessive.
• The patient recognizes that his behavior is excessive or unreasonable (this may not be true for young children or for patients whose obsessions have evolved into overvalued ideas).

Additional criteria
• At some point, the person recognizes that the obsessions or compulsions are excessive or unreasonable.
• The obsessions or compulsions cause marked distress, are time-consuming (take more than 1 hour a day), or significantly interfere with the person's normal routine, occupational functioning, or usual social activities or relationships.
• If another Axis I disorder is present, the content of the obsession is unrelated to it; for example, the ideas, thoughts, or images are not about food in the presence of an eating disorder, about drugs in the presence of a psychoactive substance abuse disorder, or about guilt thoughts in a major depressive disorder.
• The disturbance is not due to the direct physiologic effects of a substance or a general medical condition.

---

fluid intake and exhaustion. Provide for basic needs, such as rest and nutrition, if the patient becomes involved in ritualistic thoughts and behaviors to the point of self-neglect.
• Let the patient know you're aware of his behavior. For example, you might say, "I noticed you've made your bed three times today; that must be very tiring for you." Help the patient explore feelings associated with the behavior. For ex-

Behavioral therapies

The following behavioral therapies are used to treat the patient with obsessive-compulsive disorder.

Aversion therapy
Application of a painful stimulus creates an aversion to the obsession that leads to undesirable behavior (compulsion).

Thought stopping
This technique breaks the habit of fear-inducing anticipatory thoughts. The patient learns to stop unwanted thoughts by saying the word *stop* and then focusing his attention on achieving calmness and muscle relaxation.

Thought switching
To replace fear-inducing self-instructions with competent self-instructions, the patient learns to replace negative thoughts with positive ones until the positive thoughts become strong enough to overcome the anxiety-provoking ones.

Flooding
This frequent full-intensity exposure (through the use of imagery) to an object that triggers a symptom must be used with caution because it produces extreme discomfort.

Implosion therapy
A form of desensitization, implosion therapy calls for repeated exposure to a highly feared object.

Response prevention
Preventing compulsive behavior by distraction, persuasion, or redirection of activity, this form of behavior therapy may require hospitalization or involvement of the family to be effective.

---

ample, ask him, "What do you think about while you are performing your chores?"

• Make reasonable demands and set reasonable limits; make their purpose clear. Avoid creating situations that increase frustration and provoke anger, which may interfere with treatment.

• Explore patterns leading to the behavior or recurring problems. Listen attentively, offering feedback.

• Encourage the use of appropriate defense mechanisms to relieve loneliness and isolation.

• Engage the patient in activities to create positive accomplishments and raise his self-esteem and confidence.

• Encourage active diversional resources, such as whistling or humming a tune, to divert attention from the unwanted thoughts and to promote a pleasurable experience.

• Assist the patient with new ways to solve problems and to develop more effective coping skills by setting limits on unacceptable behavior (for example, by limiting the number of

times per day he may indulge in obsessive behavior). Gradually shorten the time allowed. Help him focus on other feelings or problems for the remainder of the time.
• Identify insight and improved behavior (reduced compulsive behavior and fewer obsessive thoughts). Evaluate behavioral changes by your own and the patient's reports.
• Identify disturbing topics of conversation that reflect underlying anxiety or terror.
• Observe when interventions do not work; reevaluate and recommend alternative strategies.
• Help the patient identify progress and set realistic expectations of himself and others.
• Explain how to channel emotional energy to relieve stress (for example, through sports). Also teach the patient relaxation and breathing techniques to help reduce anxiety.
• Work with the patient and other treatment team members to establish behavioral goals and to help the patient tolerate anxiety in pursuing these goals.

Posttraumatic stress disorder

Characteristic psychological consequences that persist for at least 1 month after a traumatic event outside the range of usual human experience are classified as posttraumatic stress disorder. This disorder can follow almost any distressing event: natural or man-made disaster, physical or sexual abuse, or an assault or a rape. Psychological trauma accompanies the physical trauma and involves intense fear and feelings of helplessness and loss of control. Posttraumatic stress disorder can be acute, chronic, or delayed. When the precipitating event is of human design, the disorder is more severe. Onset can occur at any age.

Causes

Posttraumatic stress disorder occurs in response to a distressing event, including a threat of harm to the patient or his family, such as war, abuse, or violent crime. It may be triggered by destruction of his home by a bombing, fire, flood, tornado, or similar disaster. It may also follow witnessing the death or serious injury of another person.

Preexisting psychopathology can predispose the patient to this disorder. However, this disorder can develop in anyone, especially if the stressor is extreme.

Signs and symptoms

The psychosocial history may reveal early life experiences, interpersonal factors, military experiences, or other incidents that suggest the precipitating event. Typically, the patient reports that his symptoms began immediately or soon after the trauma. Avoidance can prevent symptoms from developing until months or years later.

Common symptoms include pangs of painful emotion and unwelcome thoughts; intrusive memories; dissociative episodes (flashbacks); a traumatic reexperiencing of the event; difficulty falling or staying asleep, frequent nightmares of the traumatic event, and aggressive outbursts on awakening; emotional numbing—diminished or constricted response; and chronic anxiety or panic attacks.

The patient may display rage and survivor guilt; use of violence to solve problems; depression and suicidal thoughts; phobic avoidance of situations that arouse memories of trauma; memory impairment or difficulty concentrating; and feelings of detachment or estrangement that destroy interpersonal relationships. Some patients have organic symptoms, fantasies of retaliation, and substance abuse.

Diagnosis

For characteristic findings in patients with this condition, see *Diagnosing posttraumatic stress disorder.*

Treatment

Goals of treatment include reducing the target symptoms, preventing chronic disability, and promoting occupational and social rehabilitation. Specific treatment may emphasize behavioral techniques (relaxation therapy to decrease anxiety and induce sleep, or progressive desensitization); antianxiety and antidepressant drugs or psychotherapy (supportive, insight, or cathartic) to minimize the risks of dependency and chronicity.

Support groups are highly effective and are provided through many Veterans Administration centers and crisis clinics. Group settings are appropriate for most degrees of

Diagnosing posttraumatic stress disorder

The diagnosis of posttraumatic stress disorder is made when the patient's signs and symptoms meet the following criteria documented in the *DSM-IV:*
• The person was exposed to a traumatic event in which both of the following occurred:
– The person experienced, witnessed, or was confronted with an event or events that involved actual or threatened death or serious injury, or a threat to the physical integrity of self or others.
– The person's response involved intense fear, helplessness, or horror. (In children, the response may be expressed by disorganized or agitated behavior).
• The person persistently reexperiences the traumatic event in at least one of the following ways:
– recurrent and intrusive distressing recollections of the event, including images, thoughts, or perceptions
– recurrent distressing dreams of the event
– acting or feeling as if the traumatic event were recurring (includes a sense of reliving the experience, illusions, hallucinations, and dissociative episodes that occur even when awakening or intoxicated)
– intense psychological distress at exposure to internal or external cues that symbolize or resemble an aspect of the traumatic event.

• The person persistently avoids stimuli associated with the traumatic event and experiences numbing of general responsiveness (not present before the traumatic event), as indicated by at least three of the following:
– efforts to avoid thoughts or feelings associated with the trauma
– efforts to avoid activities, places, or people that arouse recollections of the trauma
– inability to recall an important aspect of the traumatic event
– markedly diminished interest in significant activities
– feeling of detachment or estrangement from other individuals
– restricted range of affect; for example, inability to love others
– sense of foreshortened future.
• The person has persistent symptoms of increased arousal (not present before the trauma), as indicated by at least two of the following:
– difficulty falling or staying asleep
– irritability or outbursts of anger
– difficulty concentrating
– hypervigilance
– exaggerated startle response.
• The disturbance must be of at least 1 month's duration.
• The disturbance causes clinically significant distress or impairment in social, occupational, or other important areas of functioning.

symptoms. Physical, social, and occupational rehabilitation programs also are available.

Many patients need treatment for depression, alcohol or drug abuse, or medical conditions before psychological healing can take place. Treatment may be complex, and the prognosis varies.

Special considerations

• Encourage the patient to express his grief, complete the mourning process, and gain coping skills to relieve anxiety and desensitize him to the memories of the traumatic event.
• Examine your feelings about the event (war or other trauma) so you won't react with disdain and shock. Reacting this way hampers the relationship with the patient and reinforces his typically poor self-image and sense of guilt.
• Practice crisis intervention techniques as appropriate.
• Accept the patient's level of functioning; assume a positive, consistent, honest, and nonjudgmental attitude.
• Provide a safe, staff-monitored room in which the patient can deal with urges to commit physical violence or self-abuse by displacement (such as pounding and throwing clay). Encourage him to move from physical to verbal expressions of anger.
• Help the patient relieve shame and guilt precipitated by actions (such as killing or mutilation) that violated a moral code. Help him put his behavior into perspective, recognize his isolation and self-destructive behavior as forms of atonement, and accept forgiveness. Refer him to clergy as appropriate.
• Provide for or refer the patient to group therapy.

Self-test questions

You can quickly review your comprehension of this chapter on anxiety disorders by answering the following questions. The correct answers to these questions and their rationales appear on pages 160 to 162.

Case history questions

David Young, age 37, has come to a phobia clinic complaining of a fear of heights. He begins to sweat, his heart pounds, he becomes short of breath, and he feels panic-stricken when confronted with heights. These symptoms have been worsening.

1. Mr. Young's history is most apt to indicate:
   a. a family history of psychiatric illness.
   b. first experiencing this fear in his late 20s.
   c. that his fear goes back to his childhood.
   d. phobias of various types in other family members.

2. Mr. Young has dealt with his phobia mainly by avoiding high places, which makes him feel:

    a. relieved.

    b. comfortable.

    c. anxious about what will happen next time.

    d. weak and ineffective.

3. The most effective treatment for Mr. Young may be:

    a. psychotherapy, as he must gain insight into the meaning of his phobia.

    b. systematic desensitization with encouragement, instruction, and suggestion.

    c. antianxiety drugs.

    d. antidepressant drugs.

Mrs. Leona Freeman, age 45, has been diagnosed with panic disorder. She has experienced exacerbations and remissions over the past 20 years. Her latest (and worst) flare-up has resulted from the death of her best friend in an auto accident.

4. Mrs. Freeman's diagnosis places her at high risk for:

    a. intense anxiety.

    b. suicide.

    c. depression.

    d. alcohol abuse.

5. If Mrs. Freeman experiences a panic attack in your presence, you can best help her by:

    a. staying with her until the attack subsides.

    b. telling her loudly that she has nothing to fear.

    c. holding her close to you.

    d. providing a complex activity to distract her.

Mr. Carl Horst repeatedly washes his hands as part of his obsessive-compulsive disorder.

6. Repeatedly washing hands:

    a. is a voluntary defense mechanism.

    b. increases his anxiety.

    c. keeps him from resorting to alcohol.
    d. reinforces recurrence of the behavior.

Jim Jones was a military frogman who served two tours of duty in Vietnam, during which many soldiers in his unit were killed or badly disabled. After returning to civilian life, he experienced posttraumatic stress disorder, demonstrating frequent nightmares, rage, and survival guilt.

7. Jim now attends a support group to allow him to:
    a. learn relaxation therapy to enhance sleep.
    b. be desensitized, reducing rage.
    c. reduce survival guilt by gaining insight through deep psychoanalysis.
    d. work through his feelings with others who've had similar conflicts.

Additional question

8. Theorists generally agree that the cause of generalized anxiety disorder is:
    a. response to an extremely distressing event.
    b. a brain lesion.
    c. conflict.
    d. reaction to danger from a particular external source.

CHAPTER 7

Somatoform Disorders

The patient with a somatoform disorder complains of physical signs and symptoms and typically travels from doctor to doctor in search of treatment. Physical examinations and laboratory tests fail to uncover an organic basis for his signs and symptoms. Somatoform disorders include somatization disorder, conversion disorder, pain disorder, and hypochondriasis.

Somatization disorder

When multiple recurrent signs and symptoms of several years' duration suggest that physical disorders exist without a verifiable disease or pathophysiologic condition to account for them, somatization disorder is present. The typical patient with somatization disorder usually undergoes repeated medical examinations and diagnostic testing that—unlike the symptoms themselves—can be potentially dangerous or debilitating. However, unlike the hypochondriac, she's not preoccupied with the belief that she has a specific disease.

Somatization disorder usually is chronic with exacerbations during times of stress. The patient's signs and symptoms are involuntary, and she consciously wants to feel better. Nonetheless, she's seldom entirely symptom-free. Onset of signs and symptoms usually occurs in adolescence or, rarely, in one's 20s. This disorder primarily affects women; it's seldom diagnosed in men.

Causes

Both genetic and environmental factors contribute to the development of somatization disorder.

Signs and
symptoms

Examination of a patient with somatization disorder is characterized by physical complaints presented in a dramatic, vague, or exaggerated way, often as part of a complicated medical history in which many physical diagnoses have been considered. An important clue to this disorder is a history of multiple medical evaluations at different institutions, with different doctors—sometimes simultaneously—without significant findings.

The patient usually appears anxious and depressed. Common physical complaints include:
• conversion or pseudoneurologic signs and symptoms (for example, paralysis or blindness)
• GI discomfort (abdominal pain, nausea, or vomiting)
• female reproductive difficulties (such as painful menstruation) or male reproductive difficulties (such as erectile dysfunction)
• psychosexual problems (for example, sexual indifference)
• chronic pain (for example, back pain)
• cardiopulmonary symptoms (chest pain, dizziness, or palpitations).

The patient with somatization disorder typically relates her current complaints and previous evaluations in great detail. She may be quite knowledgeable about tests, procedures, and medical jargon. Attempts to explore areas other than her medical history may cause noticeable anxiety. She tends to disparage previous health care professionals and previous treatment, often with the comment, "No one seems to understand. Everyone thinks I'm imagining these things."

Ongoing assessment should focus on new signs or symptoms or any change in old ones to avoid missing a developing physical disease.

Diagnosis

For characteristic findings in patients with this condition, see *Diagnosing somatization disorder.*

Diagnostic tests rule out physical disorders that cause vague and confusing somatic symptoms, such as hyperparathyroidism, porphyria, multiple sclerosis, and systemic lupus erythematosus. In addition, multiple physical signs and symptoms that appear for the first time late in life usually are due to physical disease, rather than somatization disorder.

Diagnosing somatization disorder

The diagnosis of somatization disorder is made when the patient's symptoms match the diagnostic criteria put forth in the *DSM-IV* as follows:

• A history of many physical complaints, beginning before age 30 and persisting for several years, that result in the patient seeking treatment or in the patient experiencing significant social, occupational, or other impairment.

• A selection of symptoms as follows (with individual symptoms occurring at any time during the disturbance):

— *Pain:* A history of pain related to at least *four* different sites or functions (head, abdomen, back, joints, arms and legs, chest, rectum, menstruation, sexual intercourse, or urination)

— *GI upset:* A history of at least *two* GI symptoms — other than pain (vomiting other than during pregnancy, nausea, bloating, diarrhea, intolerance of different foods)

— *Sexual symptoms:* A history of at least *one* sexual or reproductive symptom other than pain; for example, sexual indifference, erectile or ejaculatory dysfunction, irregular menses, excessive menstrual bleeding, vomiting throughout pregnancy

— *Pseudoneurologic symptom:* A history of at least *one* symptom or deficit suggesting a neurologic condition not limited to pain (for example, conversion symptoms, such as impaired coordination or balance, paralysis or localized weakness, difficulty swallowing or lump in the throat, aphonia, urine retention, hallucinations, loss of touch or pain sensation, double vision, blindness, deafness, seizures; dissociative symptoms such as amnesia; or loss of consciousness other than fainting)

• A thorough investigation discloses that either the above symptoms cannot be fully explained by a known general medical condition or the direct effects of a substance or, if a related general medical condition exists, the physical complaints or resulting impairments exceed what would be expected from the history, physical examination, or diagnostic findings.

• The symptoms are not intentionally produced or feigned (as in factitious disorder or malingering).

Treatment

The goal of treatment is to help the patient learn to live with her signs and symptoms. After diagnostic evaluation has ruled out organic causes, the patient should be told that she has no current serious illness but will receive care for her genuine distress and ongoing medical attention to her symptoms.

The most important aspect of treatment is a continuing, supportive relationship with a health care provider who acknowledges the patient's signs and symptoms and is willing to help her live with them. The patient should have regularly scheduled appointments to review her signs and symptoms and the effectiveness of her coping strategies. The patient with somatization disorder seldom acknowledges any psychological aspect of her illness and rejects psychiatric treatment.

Special
consideratons

• Acknowledge the patient's symptoms and support her efforts to function and cope despite distress. Don't characterize her signs and symptoms as imaginary. Do tell her the results and meanings of tests.
• Emphasize the patient's strengths: "It's good that you can still work with this pain." Gently point out the time relationship between stress and physical symptoms.
• Help the patient manage stress. Typically, her relationships are linked to her signs and symptoms; relieving them can impair her interactions with others.
• Negotiate your care with input from the patient and, if possible, her family. Help them to understand the patient's need for troublesome signs and symptoms.

Conversion disorder

A conversion disorder allows a patient to resolve a psychological conflict through the loss of a specific physical function – for example, by paralysis, blindness, or inability to swallow. Unlike factitious disorders or malingering, conversion disorder results in an involuntary loss of physical function (see *Factitious disorders.*) However, laboratory tests and diagnostic procedures don't disclose an organic cause. Conversion disorder can occur in either sex at any age. An uncommon disorder, it usually begins in adolescence or early in adulthood. The conversion symptom itself is not life-threatening and usually has a short duration.

Causes

The patient suddenly develops the conversion symptom soon after experiencing a traumatic conflict he believes that he cannot handle.

Signs and
symptoms

The history of a patient with conversion disorder may reveal the sudden onset of a single, debilitating sign or symptom that prevents normal function of the affected body part such as

Factitious disorders

Marked by the irrational, repetitious simulation of a physical or mental illness for the purpose of obtaining medical treatment, factitious disorders are severely psychopathologic conditions. The symptoms are intentionally produced and can be either physical or psychological. These disorders are more common in men than in women.

Factitious disorder with physical symptoms

Also called Munchausen syndrome, this is the most common factitious disorder. The patient convincingly presents with intentionally feigned symptoms. These symptoms may be fabricated (acute abdominal pain with no underlying disease), self-inflicted (deliberately infecting an open wound), an exacerbation or exaggeration of a preexisting disorder (taking penicillin despite a known allergy), or a combination of all the above.

The history of a patient with Munchausen syndrome may include:
• multiple admissions to various hospitals, typically across a wide geographic area
• extensive knowledge of medical terminology

• pathologic lying
• evidence of previous treatment such as surgery
• shifting complaints and signs and symptoms
• eagerness to undergo hazardous and painful procedures
• discharge against medical advice to avoid detection
• poor interpersonal relationships
• refusal of psychiatric examination
• psychoactive substance or analgesic use.

Factitious disorder with psychological symptoms

Causing severely impaired function, this disorder is characterized by intentional feigning of symptoms suggestive of a mental disorder. However, the symptoms represent how the patient views the mental disorder and seldom coincide with any of the diagnostic categories documented in the *DSM-IV.*

This disorder almost always coexists with a severe personality disorder. Most patients have a history of psychoactive substance use, often in an attempt to elicit the desired symptoms.

---

paralysis of a leg. The patient may describe a recent and severe psychologically stressful event that preceded the symptom. Oddly, the patient doesn't show the affect and concern that such a severe symptom usually elicits.

Assessment findings obtained during a physical examination are inconsistent with the primary symptom. For instance, tendon reflexes may be normal in a "paralyzed" part of the body, loss of function fails to follow anatomic patterns of innervation, or normal pupillary responses and evoked potentials are present in a patient who complains of blindness.

Diagnosing conversion disorder

The diagnosis of conversion disorder is based on the following criteria put forth in the *DSM-IV:*
• The person has one or more symptoms or deficits affecting voluntary motor or sensory function that suggest a neurologic or other general medical condition.
• The person exhibits psychological factors judged to be associated with the symptom or deficit because conflicts or other stressors preceded the symptom or deficit's manifestation.
• The person's symptom or deficit is not intentionally produced or feigned.
• The person's symptom or deficit can-

not, after appropriate investigation, be fully explained by a general medical condition, the direct effects of a substance, or as a culturally sanctioned behavior or experience.
• The person's symptom or deficit warrants medical evaluation, causes clinically significant distress, or impairs social, occupational, or other important areas of functioning.
• The person's symptom or deficit is not limited to pain or sexual dysfunction, does not occur exclusively during the course of somatization disorder, and is not better accounted for by another mental disorder.

Diagnosis

For characteristic findings in patients with this condition, see *Diagnosing conversion disorder.* Of course, thorough physical evaluation must rule out any physical cause, especially diseases with vague physical onsets (such as multiple sclerosis or systemic lupus erythematosus).

Treatment

Psychotherapy, family therapy, relaxation therapy, behavior therapy, or hypnosis may be used alone or in combination (two or more) to treat conversion disorder.

Special considerations

• Help the patient maintain integrity of the affected system. Regularly exercise paralyzed limbs to prevent muscle wasting and contractures.
• Frequently change the bedridden patient's position to prevent pressure ulcers.
• Ensure adequate nutrition, even if the patient is complaining of GI distress.
• Provide a supportive environment, and encourage the patient to discuss the stress that provoked the conversion disorder. Don't force the patient to talk, but convey a caring attitude to help him share his feelings.
• Don't insist that the patient use the affected system. This will only anger him and prevent a therapeutic relationship.

• Add your support to the recommendation for psychiatric care.
• Include the patient's family in all care. They may be part of the patient's stress, and they are essential to support the patient and help him regain normal functioning.

Pain disorder

The striking feature of pain disorder is a persistent complaint of pain in the absence of appropriate physical findings. The symptoms are either inconsistent with the normal anatomic distribution of the nervous system or mimic a disorder, such as angina, in the absence of diagnostic validation. Although the pain has no physical cause, it is real to the patient. The disorder is more common in women than in men and frequently has an onset in the 30s and 40s. The pain usually is chronic, often interfering with interpersonal relationships or employment.

Causes

Pain disorder has no specific cause, but it may be related to severe psychological stress or conflict. The pain provides the patient with a means to cope with upsetting psychological issues. For example, a person with dependency needs may develop this disorder as an acceptable way to receive care and attention. The pain may have special significance such as leg pain in the same leg a parent lost through amputation.

Signs and
symptoms

The cardinal feature of pain disorder is a history of chronic, consistent complaints of pain without confirming physical disease. The patient may relate a long history of evaluations and procedures at multiple settings without much pain relief. Because of frequent hospitalizations, the patient may be familiar with pain medications and tranquilizers; she may ask for a specific drug and know its correct dosage and route of administration. She may openly behave like an invalid.

Physical examination of the painful site reveals that the pain does not follow anatomic pathways. The patient may not show typical nonverbal signs of pain, such as grimacing or

Diagnosing pain disorder

The diagnosis of pain disorder is difficult because the perception of pain is subjective. According to the *DSM-IV*, diagnosis is based on fulfillment of the following criteria:

• Pain in one or more body sites is the predominant focus of the patient and is sufficiently severe to warrant clinical attention.

• The pain causes clinically significant distress or impairment in social, occupational, or other important areas of functioning.

• Psychological factors are judged to have an important role in the onset, severity, exacerbation, and maintenance of the pain.

• The symptom or deficit is not intentionally produced or feigned.

• The pain is not better accounted for by a mood, anxiety, or psychotic disorder and does not meet criteria for dyspareunia.

---

guarding. (Sometimes such reactions are absent in patients with chronic organic pain.) Palpation, percussion, and auscultation may not reveal expected associated signs. Psychosocial assessment may reveal a patient who is angry at health care professionals because they've failed to relieve her pain.

Diagnosis

For characteristic findings in patients with this condition, see *Diagnosing pain disorder.*

Treatment

In pain disorder, treatment aims to ease the pain and help the patient live with it. Thus, long, invasive evaluations and surgical interventions are avoided. Treatment at a comprehensive pain center may be helpful. Supportive measures for pain relief may include hot or cold packs, physical therapy, distraction techniques, and cutaneous stimulation with massage or transcutaneous electrical nerve stimulation. Measures to reduce the patient's anxiety may help, as may an antidepressant medication such as a tricyclic antidepressant.

A continuing, supportive relationship with an understanding health care professional is essential for effective management; regularly scheduled follow-up appointments are helpful.

Analgesics become an issue because the patient believes that she has to "fight to be taken seriously." The patient should clearly be told what medication she will receive in addition to supportive pain relief measures. Regularly scheduled analgesic doses can be more effective than scheduling medication as needed. Regular doses combat pain by reducing anxiety about asking for medication, and they eliminate unnecessary confrontations. The use of placebos will destroy trust when the patient discovers deceit.

Special considerations

• Observe and record characteristics of the pain: severity, duration, and any precipitating factors.

• Provide a caring atmosphere in which the patient's complaints are taken seriously and every effort is made to provide relief. This means communicating to the patient that you'll collaborate in a treatment plan, clearly stating the limitations. For example, you might say, "I can stay with you now for 15 minutes, but you can't receive another dose until 2 p.m."

• Don't tell the patient that she's imagining the pain or can wait longer for medication that's due. Assess her complaints and help her understand what's contributing to the pain.

• Provide other comfort measures, such as repositioning or massage, when possible.

• Encourage the patient to maintain independence despite her pain.

• Offer attention at times other than during the patient's complaints of pain, to weaken the link to secondary gain.

• Avoid confronting the patient with the somatoform nature of her pain; this seldom is helpful because such pain is her means of avoiding psychological conflict.

• Consider psychiatric referrals; however, realize that the patient may resist psychiatric intervention, and don't expect it to replace analgesic measures.

• Teach the patient noninvasive, drug-free methods of pain control, such as guided imagery, relaxation techniques, and distraction through reading or writing.

Hypochondriasis

The dominant feature of hypochondriasis is an unrealistic misinterpretation of the severity and significance of physical signs or sensations as abnormal. This leads to preoccupation with fear of having a serious disease, which persists despite medical reassurance to the contrary. Hypochondriasis causes severe social and occupational impairment. It is not due to other mental disorders, such as schizophrenia, mood disorder, or somatization disorder.

Hypochondriasis appears to be equally common in men and women. It can begin at any age, but onset most frequently occurs between ages 20 and 30. The course of the disease usually is chronic, although the severity of symptoms may vary.

Causes

Hypochondriasis is not linked to any specific cause. However, this disorder frequently develops in people or the relatives of those who have experienced an organic disease. It allows the patient to assume a dependent sick role to ensure his needs are met. Such a patient is unaware of these unmet needs and does not consciously cause his symptoms. Stress increases the risk of developing hypochondriasis.

Signs and symptoms

The dominant feature of hypochondriasis is the misinterpretation of symptoms – usually multiple complaints that involve a single organ system – as signs of serious illness. As medical evaluation proceeds, complaints may shift and change. Symptoms can range from specific to general, vague complaints, and often are associated with a preoccupation with normal body functions.

The hypochondriacal patient will relate a chronic history of waxing and waning symptoms. Commonly, he will have undergone multiple evaluations for similar symptoms or complaints of serious illness. His past contacts with health care professionals make him quite knowledgeable about illness, diagnosis, and treatment.

Diagnosis

For characteristic findings in patients with this condition, see *Diagnosing hypochondriasis.*

Diagnosing hypochondriasis

A diagnosis of hypochondriasis is made when the patient's symptoms meet the following criteria put forth in the *DSM-IV*:

• Preoccupation with the fear of having or the belief that one has a serious disease based on the person's misinterpretation of bodily symptoms.

• Preoccupation persists despite appropriate medical evaluation and reassurance.

• The fear of having or the belief that one has a serious disease is not of delusional intensity (as in delusional disorder, somatic type) and is not restricted to a circumscribed concern about appearance (as in body dysmorphic disorder).

• The preoccupation causes clinically significant distress or impairment in social, occupational, or other important areas of functioning.

• The disturbance has persisted for at least 6 months.

• The preoccupation is not better accounted for by generalized anxiety disorder, obsessive-compulsive disorder, panic disorder, a major depressive episode, separation anxiety, or another somatoform disorder.

Treatment

The goal of treatment is to help the patient continue to lead a productive life despite distressing symptoms and fears. After medical evaluation is complete, the patient should be told clearly that he doesn't have a serious disease but that continued medical follow-up will help monitor his symptoms. Providing a diagnosis won't make hypochondriasis disappear, but it may ease the patient's anxiety.

Regular outpatient follow-up can help the patient deal with his symptoms and is necessary to detect organic illness. (Up to 30% of these patients develop an organic disease.) Because the patient can be demanding and irritating, consistent follow-up may be difficult.

Most patients don't acknowledge any psychological influence on their symptoms and resist psychiatric treatment.

Special considerations

• Provide a supportive relationship that lets the patient feel cared for and understood. The patient with hypochondriasis feels real pain and distress, so don't deny his symptoms or challenge his behavior.

• Firmly state that medical test results were negative. Instead of reinforcing his symptoms, encourage him to discuss his other problems, and urge his family to do the same.

• Recognize that the patient will never be symptom-free, and don't become angry when he won't give up his disease. Such anger can drive the patient away to yet another unnecessary medical evaluation.

• Help the patient and family find new ways to deal with stress other than development of physical symptoms. For example, teaching the patient more effective coping strategies can reduce his need to resort to hypochondriacal behavior.

Self-test questions

You can quickly review your comprehension of this chapter on somatoform disorders by answering the following questions. The correct answers to these questions and their rationales appear on pages 162 and 163.

Case history questions

Mary Novak, age 42, has been diagnosed with somatization disorder after years of diagnostic testing and multiple consultations for vague GI and reproductive difficulties.

1. While under your care, Mrs. Novak will require ongoing evaluation for new signs and symptoms and for any change in old ones to:
   a. be certain a verifiable disease hasn't been present all along.
   b. avoid missing a developing physical disease.
   c. investigate her anxiety or depression.
   d. ensure that she isn't malingering.

2. The most important aspect of Mrs. Novak's treatment is:
   a. relieving her signs and symptoms.
   b. reducing her anxiety.
   c. convincing her of the importance of participating in psychiatric treatment.
   d. ongoing support from her chief caregiver.

The Reverend David Ralphson has suddenly lost the ability to speak. Diagnostic studies ruled out an organic cause, and conversion disorder was diagnosed.

3. Rev. Ralphson's loss of physical function is considered to be:
    a. involuntary.
    b. voluntary.
    c. factitious.
    d. malingering.

4. An important part of Rev. Ralphson's care will be:
    a. asking him to use his voice, perhaps to sing.
    b. repeatedly reminding him that his inability to speak has no physical cause.
    c. helping him maintain the integrity of vocal muscles through prescribed exercises.
    d. insisting that he try to speak and placing him in situations requiring him to speak.

Rosa Gonzalez was recently diagnosed with pain disorder and supportive analgesic measures haven't controlled her pain. She will need medication.

5. When pain disorders require medication in addition to supportive measures, be sure to:
    a. tell the patient an analgesic will be prescribed without giving specific drug information.
    b. administer the drug as needed.
    c. use a placebo to help determine whether or not the pain is real.
    d. administer the drug in regularly scheduled doses.

Eva Simpson is being treated for hypochondriasis.

6. One risk factor for hypochondriasis is:
    a. aging.
    b. another mental disorder.
    c. stress.
    d. being female.

7. Mrs. Simpson demonstrates typical hypochondriacal behaviors in that she:

    a. knowingly assumes a sick role to meet her dependency needs.

    b. is unaware of her unmet needs and isn't consciously causing her symptoms.

    c. recognizes her unmet needs but doesn't know a healthful way to resolve them.

    d. is preoccupied with the size and shape of her bust, hips, and legs.

8. When caring for Mrs. Simpson, you should:

    a. help her to give up her disease.

    b. challenge her symptoms.

    c. treat and remove her symptoms.

    d. recognize that she will never be symptom-free.

CHAPTER 8

Dissociative and Personality Disorders

"Dissociation" refers to an unconscious defense mechanism that keeps troubling thoughts out of a person's awareness. The patient with a dissociative disorder experiences temporary changes in consciousness, identity, and motor function. The patient with a personality disorder suffers chronic, maladaptive behavior patterns. The disorders included in this section are dissociative identity disorder, dissociative fugue, dissociative amnesia, depersonalization disorder, and personality disorders.

Dissociative identity disorder

A complex disturbance of identity and memory, dissociative identity disorder (formerly referred to as "multiple personality disorder") is characterized by the existence of two or more distinct, fully integrated personalities in the same person. The personalities alternate in dominance. Each comprises unique memories, behavior patterns, and social relationships; rigid and flamboyant personalities often are combined. Usually, one personality is unaware of the existence of the others.

Dissociative identity disorder usually begins in childhood, but patients seldom seek treatment until much later in life. The disorder is three to nine times more common in women than in men.

Diagnosing dissociative identity disorder

The diagnosis of dissociative identity disorder is based on fulfillment of the following criteria established in the *DSM-IV*:

• Two or more distinct personalities or personality states (each with its own relatively enduring pattern of perceiving, relating to, and thinking about the environment and self) are present.

• At least two of these personalities or personality states recurrently take full control of the person's behavior.

• The person cannot recall important personal information that is too extensive to be explained by ordinary forgetfulness.

• The disturbance is not due to the direct physiologic effects of a substance or a general medical condition.

Causes

The cause of dissociative identity disorder is not known. The patient typically has experienced abuse, often sexual, or another form of severe emotional trauma in childhood. Psychiatrists believe that a child exposed to such overwhelming stimuli may evolve multiple personalities to dissociate herself from the traumatic situation. The dissociated contents become linked with one of many possible shaping influences for personality organization.

Signs and symptoms

The patient with dissociative identity disorder may seek medical treatment for a concurrent psychiatric disorder, present in one of the personalities. She may have a history of unsuccessful psychiatric treatment, or she may report periods of amnesia and disturbances in time perception. Family members or friends may describe incidents that the patient can't recall as well as pronounced alterations in facial presentation, voice, and behavior.

The transition from one personality to another often is triggered by stress or idiosyncratically meaningful social or environmental cues. Although usually sudden (seconds to minutes), the transition can occur over hours or days. Hypnosis and amobarbital may facilitate transition.

Diagnosis

For characteristic findings in patients with this condition, see *Diagnosing dissociative identity disorder*.

Treatment

Psychotherapy is essential to uniting the personalities and preventing the personality from splitting again. Treatment is usually intensive and prolonged, with success linked to the

strength of the patient-therapist relationship with each of the personalities. All of the personalities, whether disagreeable or congenial, require equal respect and empathetic concern.

Special considerations
• Establish an empathetic relationship with each emerging personality.
• Monitor the patient's actions for evidence of self-directed violence or violence directed at others.
• Recognize even small gains.
• Stress the importance of continuing psychotherapy. Point out that the therapy can be prolonged, with alternating successes and failures, and that one or more of the personalities may resist treatment.

Dissociative fugue

The patient suffering from dissociative fugue wanders or travels while mentally blocking out a traumatic event. During the fugue state, he usually assumes a different personality and later can't recall what happened. The degree of impairment varies, depending on the duration of the fugue and the nature of the personality state it invokes. Dissociative fugue may be related to dissociative identity disorder, narcissistic personality disorder, and sleepwalking.

The age of onset varies. Although the fugue state usually is brief (hours to days), it can last for many months and carry the patient far from home. The prognosis is good for complete recovery, and recurrences are rare.

Causes
Dissociative fugue typically follows an extremely stressful event, such as combat experience, a natural disaster, a violent or abusive confrontation, or personal rejection. Heavy alcohol use may constitute a predisposing factor.

Signs and symptoms
Psychiatric examination of the patient with dissociative fugue may reveal that he's assumed a new, more uninhibited identity. If the new personality is still evolving, he may avoid

Diagnosing dissociative fugue

The diagnosis of dissociative fugue is made when the patient's symptoms match the following criteria put forth in the *DSM-IV:*
• The predominant disturbance is sudden, unexpected travel away from home or the patient's customary place of work, with an inability to recall the past.
• The person experiences confusion about personal identity or assumption of a new partial or complete identity.

• The disturbance is not due to dissociative identity disorder, physiologic effects of a substance, or a general medical condition.
• The symptoms cause clinically significant distress or impairment in social, occupational, or other important areas of functioning.

social contact. On the other hand, he may have traveled to a distant location, set up a new residence, and developed a well-integrated network of social relationships that don't suggest any mental alteration.

The psychosocial history of such a patient may include episodes of violent behavior. After recovery, he typically can't remember these and other events that took place during the fugue state.

Diagnosis

For characteristic findings in patients with this condition, see *Diagnosing dissociative fugue.*

Treatment

Psychotherapy aims to help the patient recognize the traumatic event that triggered the fugue state and to develop reality-based strategies for coping with anxiety. A trusting, therapeutic relationship is essential for successful therapy.

Special considerations

• Assist the patient in using reality-based coping strategies under stress, rather than those strategies that distort reality.
• Help the patient recognize and deal with anxiety-producing experiences.
• Establish a therapeutic, nonjudgmental relationship.
• Teach the patient effective coping strategies to use in stressful situations, rather than those strategies that distort reality.

Types of amnesia

The *DSM-IV* recognizes five types of amnesia, based on the time period and amount of information lost to recall:
• *Localized amnesia*—failure to recall all events that occurred during a circumscribed time period
• *Selective amnesia*—failure to recall some of the events that occurred during a circumscribed time period

• *Generalized amnesia*—failure to recall all events over the entire life span
• *Continuous amnesia*—failure to recall events subsequent to a specific time up to and including the present
• *Systematized amnesia*—failure to recall certain categories of information.

Dissociative amnesia

The essential feature of dissociative amnesia is a sudden inability to recall important personal information that cannot be explained by ordinary forgetfulness. The patient typically is unable to recall all events that occurred during a specific time period, but other types of recall disturbance also are possible. (See *Types of amnesia.*)

This disorder commonly occurs during war and natural disasters. Although it is more common in adolescents and young adult women, it also is seen in young men after combat experience. The amnesic event typically ends abruptly, and recovery is complete, with rare recurrences.

Causes

Dissociative amnesia follows severe psychosocial stress, often involving a threat of physical injury or death. Amnesia also may occur after thinking about or engaging in unacceptable behavior such as an extramarital affair.

Signs and symptoms

During the assessment interview, the amnesic patient may appear perplexed and disoriented, wandering aimlessly. He won't be able to remember the event that precipitated the episode and probably won't recognize his inability to recall information.

After the episode has ended, the patient usually is unaware that he has suffered what is known as a recall disturbance.

Diagnosing dissociative amnesia

A diagnosis of dissociative amnesia is made when the patient's symptoms meet the following criteria put forth in the *DSM-IV:*
• The predominant disturbance is at least one episode of inability to recall important personal information, usually of a traumatic or stressful nature, that is too extensive to be explained by ordinary forgetfulness.

• The disturbance is not due to dissociative identity disorder, dissociative fugue, posttraumatic stress disorder, acute stress disorder, or somatization disorder and is not due to the direct physiologic effects of a substance or a neurologic or other general medical condition.
• The symptoms cause clinically significant distress or impairment in social, occupational, or other important areas of functioning.

Diagnosis

For characteristic findings in patients with this condition, see *Diagnosing dissociative amnesia.*

Treatment

Psychotherapy aims to help the patient recognize the traumatic event that triggered the amnesia and the anxiety it produced. A trusting therapeutic relationship is essential to achieving this goal. The therapist subsequently attempts to teach the patient reality-based coping strategies.

Special considerations

• Assist the patient in using reality-based coping strategies under stress, rather than those strategies that distort reality.
• Help the patient recognize and deal with anxiety-producing experiences.
• Establish a therapeutic, nonjudgmental relationship.
• Teach the patient effective coping strategies to use in stressful situations, rather than those strategies that distort reality.

Depersonalization disorder

Persistent or recurrent episodes of detachment characterize depersonalization disorder. During these episodes, self-awareness is temporarily altered or lost; the patient often perceives this alteration in consciousness as a barrier be-

Diagnosing depersonalization disorder

The depersonalization disorder diagnosis is made when the patient's symptoms match the following criteria in the *DSM-IV:*

• Persistent or recurrent experiences of feeling detached from mind or body (as if the person were an outside observer) or feeling like an automaton (as if the person were in a dream).
• During the depersonalization experience reality testing remains intact.

• The depersonalization disorder causes clinically significant distress or impairment in social, occupational, or other important areas of functioning.
• The depersonalization experience does not occur exclusively during the course of another mental disorder, such as schizophrenia, panic disorder, acute stress disorder, or another dissociative disorder, and is not due to the direct physiologic effects of a substance or a general medical condition.

tween himself and the outside world. The sense of depersonalization may be restricted to a single body part, such as a limb, or it may encompass the whole self.

Although the patient seldom loses touch with reality completely, the episodes of depersonalization may cause him severe distress. Depersonalization disorder usually has a sudden onset in adolescence or early in adult life. It follows a chronic course, with periodic exacerbations and remissions, and resolves gradually.

Causes

Depersonalization disorder typically stems from severe stress, including war experiences, accidents, and natural disasters.

Signs and symptoms

The patient with depersonalization disorder may complain of feeling detached from his entire being and body, as if he were watching himself from a distance or living in a dream. He also may report sensory anesthesia, a loss of self-control, difficulty speaking, and feelings of derealization.

Common findings during the assessment interview include symptoms of depression, obsessive rumination, somatic concerns, anxiety, fear of going insane, a disturbed sense of time, and a prolonged recall time, as well as physical complaints such as dizziness.

Diagnosis

For characteristic findings in patients with this condition, see *Diagnosing depersonalization disorder.*

Treatment

Psychotherapy aims to establish a trusting therapeutic relationship in which the patient recognizes the traumatic event and the anxiety it evoked. The therapist subsequently teaches the patient to use reality-based coping strategies, rather than to detach himself from the situation.

Special considerations

• Assist the patient in using reality-based coping strategies under stress, rather than those strategies that distort reality.
• Help the patient recognize and deal with anxiety-producing experiences.
• Establish a therapeutic, nonjudgmental relationship.
• Teach the patient effective coping strategies to use in stressful situations, rather than those strategies that distort reality.

Personality disorders

Defined as individual traits that reflect chronic, inflexible, and maladaptive patterns of behavior, personality disorders cause social discomfort and impair social and occupational functioning. Although no statistics exist to quantify personality disorders, they are, nevertheless, widespread. Most patients with personality disorders don't receive treatment; when they do, they're typically managed as outpatients.

Personality disorders fall on Axis II of the *Diagnostic and Statistical Manual of Mental Disorders,* 4th edition *(DSM-IV)* classification. Personality notations are appropriate and useful for all patients and help give a fuller picture of the patient and a more accurate diagnosis. For example, many features characteristic of personality disorders are apparent during an episode of another mental disorder (such as a major depressive episode in a patient with compulsive personality features).

The prognosis is variable. Personality disorders typically have an onset before or during adolescence and early adulthood and persist throughout adult life.

Causes

Only recently have personality disorders been categorized in detail, and research continues to identify their causes.

Various theories attempt to explain the origin of personality disorders. Biological theories hold that these disorders may stem from chromosomal and neuronal abnormalities or head trauma. Social theories hold that the disorders reflect learned responses, having much to do with reinforcement, modeling, and aversive stimuli as contributing factors. Psychodynamic theories hold that personality disorders reflect deficiencies in ego and superego development and are related to poor mother-child relationships that are fraught with unresponsiveness, overprotectiveness, or early separation.

Signs and symptoms

Each specific personality disorder produces characteristic signs and symptoms, which may vary among patients and within the same patient at different times. In general, the history of the patient with a personality disorder will reveal long-standing difficulties in interpersonal relations, ranging from dependency to withdrawal, and in occupational functioning, with effects ranging from compulsive perfectionism to intentional sabotage.

The patient with a personality disorder may show any degree of self-confidence ranging from no self-esteem to arrogance. Convinced that his behavior is normal, he avoids responsibility for the consequences of his behavior, often resorting to projections and blame.

Diagnosis

For characteristic findings in patients with this condition, see *Diagnosing personality disorders,* pages 130 to 133.

Treatment

Personality disorders are difficult to treat. Therapy depends on the patient's symptoms but requires a trusting relationship in which the therapist can use a direct approach.

Drug therapy is ineffective but may be used to relieve severe distress, such as acute anxiety and depression. Family and group therapy usually are effective.

Hospital inpatient milieu therapy in crisis situations and possibly for long-term treatment of borderline personality disorders can be effective. Inpatient treatment is controversial, however, because most patients with personality disorders are noncompliant with extended therapeutic regimens; for such patients, outpatient therapy may be more useful.

(Text continues on page 134.)

Diagnosing personality disorders

The diagnosis of a recognized personality disorder is made when a patient's symptoms match the following relevant diagnostic criteria put forth in the *DSM-IV.*

Paranoid personality disorder
• The person must exhibit a pervasive and unwarranted tendency, beginning by early adulthood and present in various contexts, to interpret the actions of people as deliberately demeaning or threatening as indicated by at least four of the following:
—The person suspects, without sufficient basis, that he's being exploited, deceived, or harmed by others.
—The person questions without justification the loyalty or trustworthiness of friends or associates.
—The person is reluctant to confide in others because of unwarranted fear that the information will be used against him.
—The person finds hostile or evil meanings in benign remarks.
—The person bears grudges or is unforgiving of insults or slights.
—The person is easily slighted and quick to react with anger or to counterattack.
—The person questions without justification the fidelity of a spouse or sexual partner.
• The symptoms do not occur exclusively during the course of schizophrenia or other psychotic disorders and are not the direct physiologic effect of a general medical condition.

Schizoid personality disorder
• The patient must exhibit a pervasive pattern of indifference to social relationships and a restricted range of emotional experience and expression, beginning by early adulthood and present in various contexts, as indicated by at least four of the following:
—The person neither desires nor enjoys close relationships, including being part of a family.
—The person almost always chooses solitary activities.
—The person seldom, if ever, claims or appears to experience strong emotions, such as anger and joy.
—The person indicates little, if any, desire to have sexual experiences with another person.
—The person is indifferent to the praise and criticism of others.
—The person has no close friends or confidants other than first-degree relatives.
—The person displays flat affect.
• The symptoms do not occur exclusively during the course of schizophrenia, another psychotic disorder, or a pervasive developmental disorder and are not the direct physiologic effect of a general medical condition.

Schizotypal personality disorder
• This pervasive pattern of social and interpersonal deficits is marked by acute discomfort with, and reduced capacity for, close relationships as well as by cognitive or perceptual distortions and eccentricities of behavior, beginning by early adulthood and present in various contexts. The person with schizotypal personality disorder has at least five of the following:
—ideas of reference (excluding delusions of reference)
—odd beliefs or magical thinking, influencing behavior and inconsistent with subcultural norms

Diagnosing personality disorders *(continued)*

— unusual perceptual experiences, including bodily illusions
— odd thinking and speech
— suspiciousness or paranoid thinking
— inappropriate or flat affect
— odd behavior or appearance
— no close friends or confidants other than first-degree relatives
— excessive social anxiety that does not diminish with familiarity and tends to be associated with paranoid fears rather than negative self-judgment.
• The symptoms do not occur exclusively during the course of schizophrenia, a mood disorder with psychotic features, another psychotic disorder, or a pervasive developmental disorder.

Antisocial personality disorder
• This disorder manifests as a pervasive disregard for and violation of the rights of others occurring since age 15, as indicated by at least three of the following:
— The person fails to conform to social norms with respect to lawful behavior, as demonstrated by repeatedly performing acts that are grounds for arrest.
— The person exhibits deceitfulness, as indicated by repeated lying, using aliases, or conning others for personal profit or pleasure.
— The person demonstrates impulsivity or failure to plan ahead.
— The person is irritable and aggressive, as indicated by repeated physical fights or assaults.
— The person has reckless disregard for the safety of self or others.
— The person shows consistent irresponsibility, as indicated by repeated failure to sustain consistent work behavior or honor financial obligations.
— The person lacks remorse, as indicated by being indifferent to or rational-

izing having hurt, mistreated, or stolen from others.
• The person is at least age 18.
• The person's history includes evidence of a conduct disorder with onset before age 15.
• The antisocial behavior does not occur exclusively during the course of schizophrenia or a manic episode.

Borderline personality disorder
This pervasive pattern of instability of interpersonal relationships, self-image and affect, and marked impulsivity, beginning by early adulthood and present in various contexts, is indicated by at least five of the following features:
• The person makes frantic efforts to avoid real or imagined abandonment (excluding suicidal or self-mutilating behavior).
• The person has a pattern of unstable and intense interpersonal relationships characterized by alternating between extremes of overidealization and devaluation.
• The person has an identity disturbance—a markedly and persistently unstable self-image or sense of self.
• The person shows impulsiveness in at least two areas that are potentially self-damaging, such as spending, sexual activity, substance abuse, shoplifting, reckless driving, and binge eating (excluding suicidal or self-mutilating behavior).
• The person engages in recurrent suicidal threats, gestures, or behavior, or self-mutilating behavior.
• The person has affective instability resulting from marked mood reactivity (for example, depression, irritability, or anxiety, lasting usually a few hours and seldom more than a few days).

(continued)

Diagnosing personality disorders *(continued)*

• The person has chronic feelings of emptiness or boredom.
• The person has inappropriate, intense anger or difficulty controlling anger.
• The person has transient, stress-related paranoid ideation or severe dissociative symptoms.

Histrionic personality disorder
This pervasive pattern of excessive emotionality and attention-seeking behavior, beginning by early adulthood and present in various contexts, is indicated by at least four of the following:
• The person is uncomfortable in situations in which he is not the center of attention.
• The person's interaction with others is often characterized by inappropriately sexually seductive or provocative behavior.
• The person displays rapidly shifting and shallow expression of emotions.
• The person consistently uses physical appearance to draw attention to self.
• The person has a style of speech that is excessively impressionistic and lacking in detail.
• The person shows self-dramatization, theatricality, and exaggerated emotional expression.
• The person is suggestible (easily influenced by others or circumstances).
• The person considers relationships to be more intimate than they actually are.

Narcissistic personality disorder
This pervasive pattern of grandiosity, need for admiration, and lack of empathy, beginning by early adulthood and present in various contexts, is indicated by at least five of the following:
• The person has a grandiose sense of self-importance.

• The person is preoccupied with fantasies of unlimited success, power, brilliance, beauty, or ideal love.
• The person believes that he is "special" and unique and can only be understood by, or should associate with, other special or high-status people (or institutions).
• The person requires excessive admiration.
• The person has a sense of entitlement (unreasonable expectation of especially favorable treatment or automatic compliance with his expectations).
• The person is interpersonally exploitive, taking advantage of others to achieve his own ends.
• The person lacks empathy.
• The person is often envious of others or believes that others are envious of him.
• The person shows arrogant, haughty behaviors or attitudes.

Avoidant personality disorder
This pervasive pattern of social inhibition, feelings of inadequacy, and hypersensitivity to negative evaluation, beginning by early adulthood and present in a variety of contexts, is indicated by at least four of the following:
• The person avoids social or occupational activities that involve significant interpersonal contact because of fears of criticism, disapproval, or rejection.
• The person is unwilling to get involved with people unless he's certain that they will like him.
• The person shows restraint within intimate relationships because of the fear of being shamed or ridiculed.
• The person is preoccupied with being criticized or rejected in social situations.
• The person's feelings of inadequacy inhibit him in new interpersonal situations.

Diagnosing personality disorders *(continued)*

• The person views himself as socially inept, personally unappealing, or inferior to others.

• The person is unusually reluctant to take personal risks or to engage in any new activities because they may prove embarrassing.

Dependent personality disorder

This pervasive and excessive need to be taken care of that leads to submissive and clinging behavior and fears of separation, beginning by early adulthood and present in a variety of contexts, is indicated by at least five of the following:

• The person has difficulty making everyday decisions without an excessive amount of advice or reassurance from others.

• The person needs others to assume responsibility for most major areas of his life.

• The person has difficulty expressing disagreement with others because of fear of loss of support or approval (excluding realistic fears of retribution).

• The person has difficulty initiating projects or doing things on his own (because of a lack of self-confidence in judgment or abilities rather than a lack of motivation or energy).

• The person goes to excessive lengths to obtain nurture and support from others, to the point of volunteering to do things that are unpleasant.

• The person feels uncomfortable or helpless when alone because of exaggerated fears of inability to care for himself.

• The person urgently seeks another relationship as a source of care and support when a close relationship ends.

• The person is unrealistically preoccupied with fears of being left to take care of himself.

Obsessive-compulsive personality disorder

This pervasive pattern of preoccupation with orderliness, perfectionism, and mental and interpersonal control, at the expense of flexibility, openness, and efficiency, beginning by early adulthood and present in a variety of contexts, is indicated by at least four of the following:

• The person is preoccupied with details, rules, lists, order, organization, or schedules to the extent that the core point of the activity is lost.

• The person shows perfectionism that interferes with task completion.

• The person is excessively devoted to work and productivity to the exclusion of leisure activities and friendships (not accounted for by obvious economic need).

• The person exhibits overconscientiousness, scrupulousness, and inflexibility about matters of morality, ethics, or values (not accounted for by cultural or religious identification).

• The person cannot discard worn-out or worthless objects even when they have no sentimental value.

• The person is reluctant to delegate tasks or to work with others unless they submit exactly to his way of doing things.

• The person adopts a miserly spending style toward self and others; money is viewed as something to be hoarded for future catastrophes.

• The person shows rigidity and stubbornness.

Special
considerations

• Provide consistent care. Take a direct, involved approach to ensure the patient's trust. Keep in mind that many of these patients don't respond well to interviewing, whereas others are charming and convincing.
• Teach the patient social skills, and reinforce appropriate behavior.
• Encourage expression of feelings, self-analysis of behavior, and accountability for actions.

Specific care measures vary with the particular personality disorder.

For paranoid personality disorder

• Avoid situations that threaten the patient's autonomy.
• Approach the patient in a straightforward and candid manner. Make sure to adopt a professional, rather than a casual or friendly, attitude. Remember that remarks that you intend to be humorous are easily misinterpreted by the paranoid patient.
• Provide a supportive and nonjudgmental environment in which the patient can safely explore and verbalize his feelings.

For schizoid personality disorder

• Remember that the schizoid patient needs close human contact but is easily overwhelmed. Respect the patient's need for privacy, and slowly build a trusting therapeutic relationship so that he finds more pleasure than fear in relating to you.
• Give the patient plenty of time to express his feelings. Keep in mind that if you push him to do so before he's ready, he may retreat.

For schizotypal personality disorder

• Recognize that this type of patient is easily overwhelmed by stress. Allow him plenty of time to make difficult decisions.
• Be aware that the patient may relate unusually well to certain staff members and not at all to others.

For antisocial personality disorder

• Be clear about your expectations and the consequences of failing to meet them.
• Use a straightforward, matter-of-fact approach to set limits on unacceptable behavior. Encourage and reinforce positive behavior.
• Expect the patient to refuse to cooperate so that he can gain control.

For borderline personality disorder

- Encourage the patient to take responsibility for himself. Don't attempt to rescue him from the consequences of his actions.
- Don't try to solve problems that the patient can solve himself.
- Maintain a consistent approach in all interactions with the patient; ensure that other team members use the same approach.
- Recognize that the patient may idolize some staff members and devalue others.
- Don't take sides in the patient's disputes with other staff members.

For histrionic personality disorder

- Give the patient choices in care strategies, and incorporate his wishes into the treatment plan as much as possible. By increasing the patient's sense of self-control, you'll reduce his anxiety.
- Approach the patient formally. He may be uncomfortable with a casual approach.

For narcissistic personality disorder

- Respond positively to the patient's sense of entitlement. A critical attitude may cause him to become even more demanding and difficult.
- Focus on positive traits or on his feelings of pain, loss, or rejection.

For avoidant personality disorder

- Assess the patient for signs of depression. Social impairment increases the risk of affective disorders in these patients with avoidant personality disorder.
- Establish a trusting interpersonal relationship with the patient. Be aware that he may become dependent on the few staff members whom he believes he can trust.
- Make sure that all upcoming procedures are known to the patient in plenty of time for him to adjust. This patient is unable to handle surprises well.
- Inform the patient when you will and will not be available if he needs assistance.

For dependent personality disorder

- Initially, give the patient explicit directives, rather than ask him to make decisions. Then encourage him to make easy decisions, such as what to wear or which television program to watch. Continue to provide the patient with support and reassurance as his decision-making ability improves.

For obsessive-compulsive personality disorder

• Allow the patient to participate in his own treatment plan by offering choices whenever possible.
• Adopt a professional approach in your interactions with the patient. Avoid informality; this patient expects strict attention to detail.

Self-test questions

You can quickly review your comprehension of this chapter on dissociative and personality disorders by answering the following questions. The correct answers to these questions and their rationales appear on pages 164 and 165.

Case history questions

Ashley Waters, a doctoral student who was sexually and emotionally abused as a child, sought medical help because she experienced periods of amnesia and disturbances in time perception. Dissociative identity disorder has been diagnosed.

1. Dissociative identity disorder is characterized by:
   a. the existence of more than one distinct and fully integrated personality in the same person.
   b. wandering or traveling while assuming a different personality and later not recalling what happened.
   c. sudden inability to recall important personal information that can't be explained by ordinary forgetfulness.
   d. inability to recall all events that occurred during a specific time period.

2. Ashley usually is a rather rigid, quiet, and restrained young woman, but friends at school report occasional outbursts of a very different Ashley: a flamboyant, outgoing, "party girl," who uses suggestive language and postures. Finding risqué outfits in her closet, Ashley would most likely assume that:

a. they belong to a friend who visited at a time she can't remember.
b. they belong to her other personality.
c. she must have bought them to give to someone else.
d. they were planted in her closet by someone who wishes her ill.

3. Treatment to unite Ashley's personalities will involve:
a. behavior modification therapy.
b. intensive psychotherapy.
c. use of psychotropic drugs.
d. use of anxiolytic drugs.

Joe Callahan has been diagnosed with dissociative fugue. Calling himself Jim Baker, Mr. Callahan traveled to Florida, established new relationships, and found a job as a waiter in a diner. He was discovered when police officers recognized him as a missing person when they stopped in the diner for breakfast.

4. In dissociative fugue, the fugue state usually lasts:
a. hours to days.
b. days to weeks.
c. weeks to months.
d. months to years.

5. Typically, dissociative fugue follows:
a. a long period of unhappiness.
b. a routine family disagreement.
c. intermittent bouts of depression.
d. extreme stress.

Mona Tisdale, age 21, has a tendency to drink heavily. Recently, she survived a serious fire in San Francisco, but both her parents died in the disaster. In the days following the fire, Mona appeared disoriented and couldn't recall anything about the episode. She was diagnosed with dissociative amnesia.

6. Dissociative amnesia commonly occurs:
   a. after heavy alcohol use.
   b. with use of psychotropic drugs.
   c. during war and natural disasters.
   d. with severe physical injury.

Nancy Thomas, age 27, has suffered from depersonalization disorder for the last 10 years.

7. Nancy complains of:
   a. feeling the need for rigid self-control.
   b. feeling detached from her body.
   c. having frequent nightmares and bad dreams.
   d. feeling the need to talk continually.

8. A common finding in depersonalization disorder is:
   a. fear of going insane.
   b. disorientation to place.
   c. absence of physical complaints.
   d. inability to recall past personal history.

CHAPTER 9

Eating Disorders

The disorders in this section include bulimia nervosa and anorexia nervosa, which mainly affect adolescents.

Bulimia nervosa

The essential features of bulimia nervosa include eating binges followed by feelings of guilt, humiliation, and self-deprecation. These feelings precipitate the patient's engaging in self-induced vomiting, the use of laxatives or diuretics, or strict dieting or fasting to overcome the effects of the binges. Unless the patient devotes an excessive amount of time to binging and purging, bulimia nervosa seldom is incapacitating. However, electrolyte imbalances (including metabolic alkalosis, hypochloremia, and hypokalemia) and dehydration can occur, increasing the risk of serious physical complications.

Bulimia nervosa usually begins in adolescence or early adulthood and can occur simultaneously with anorexia nervosa. It affects nine women for every one man. Nearly 2% of adult women meet the diagnostic criteria for bulimia nervosa; 5% to 15% have some symptoms of the disorder.

Causes

The exact cause of bulimia is unknown, but various psychosocial factors are thought to contribute to its development. Such factors include family disturbance or conflict, sexual abuse, maladaptive learned behavior, struggle for control or self-identity, cultural overemphasis on physical appearance, and parental obesity. Bulimia nervosa is strongly associated with depression.

Signs and symptoms

The history of a patient with bulimia nervosa is characterized by episodes of binge eating that may occur up to sev-

Characteristics of bulimic patients

Recognizing the bulimic patient isn't always easy. Unlike anorexic patients, bulimic patients don't deny that their eating habits are abnormal, but they commonly conceal their behavior out of shame and humiliation. If you suspect bulimia nervosa, be on the lookout for the following features:
• difficulty with impulse control
• chronic depression
• exaggerated sense of guilt
• low tolerance for frustration
• recurrent anxiety
• feelings of alienation
• self-consciousness
• difficulty expressing feelings such as anger
• impaired social or occupational adjustment.

eral times a day. The patient commonly reports a binge-eating episode during which she continues eating until abdominal pain, sleep, or the presence of another person interrupts it. The preferred food usually is sweet, soft, and high in calories and carbohydrate content.

The bulimic patient may appear thin and emaciated. Typically, however, although the patient's weight frequently fluctuates, it usually stays within the normal range—through the use of diuretics, laxatives, vomiting, and exercise. So, unlike the anorexic patient, the bulimic patient usually can keep her eating disorder hidden.

Overt clues to this disorder include hyperactivity, peculiar eating habits or rituals, frequent weighing, and a distorted body image. (See *Characteristics of bulimic patients*.)

The patient may complain of abdominal and epigastric pain caused by acute gastric dilation. She may also have amenorrhea. Repetitive vomiting may cause painless swelling of the salivary glands, hoarseness, throat irritation or lacerations, and dental erosion. In addition, the patient may exhibit calluses of the knuckles or abrasions and scars on the dorsum of the hand, resulting from tooth injury during self-induced vomiting.

A bulimic patient commonly is perceived by others as a "perfect" student, mother, or career woman; an adolescent may be distinguished for participation in competitive activities, such as gymnastics, sports, or ballet. However, the patient's psychosocial history may reveal an exaggerated sense of guilt, symptoms of depression, childhood trauma (espe-

Diagnosing bulimia nervosa

The diagnosis of bulimia is made when the patient meets criteria put forth in the *DSM-IV.* Both of the behaviors listed below must occur at least twice a week for 3 months:
• recurrent episodes of binge eating (rapid consumption of a large amount of food in a discrete period of time and a feeling of lack of control over eating behavior during the eating binges)
• recurrent inappropriate compensatory behavior to prevent weight gain (self-induced vomiting; misuse of laxatives, diuretics, enemas, or other medications; fasting; excessive exercise).

---

cially sexual abuse), parental obesity, or a history of unsatisfactory sexual relationships.

Diagnosis

For characteristic findings in patients with this condition, see *Diagnosing bulimia nervosa.*

Additional diagnostic tools include the Beck Depression Inventory, which may identify coexisting depression. And laboratory tests can help determine the presence and severity of complications. Serum electrolyte studies may show elevated bicarbonate, decreased potassium, and decreased sodium levels.

A baseline electrocardiogram may be done if tricyclic antidepressants will be prescribed for the patient.

Treatment

Therapy for bulimia nervosa may continue for several years. Interrelated physical and psychological symptoms must be treated simultaneously. Merely promoting weight gain isn't sufficient to guarantee long-term recovery. A patient whose physical status is severely compromised by inadequate or chaotic eating patterns is difficult to engage in the psychotherapeutic process.

Psychotherapy concentrates on interrupting the binge-purge cycle and helping the patient regain control over her eating behavior. Treatment may be provided in either an inpatient or outpatient setting and includes behavior modification therapy, possibly in highly structured psychoeducational group meetings. Individual psychotherapy and family therapy, which address the eating disorder as a symptom of unresolved conflict, may help the patient understand the basis of her behavior and teach her self-control strategies. Antidepressant drugs may be used as an adjunct to psychotherapy.

The patient also may benefit from participation in self-help groups, such as Overeaters Anonymous, or in a drug rehabilitation program if she has a concurrent substance abuse problem.

Special considerations

• Supervise the patient during mealtimes and for a specified period after meals (usually 1 hour). Set a time limit for each meal. Provide a pleasant, relaxed environment for eating.

• Using behavior modification techniques, reward the patient for satisfactory weight gain.

• Establish a contract with the patient, specifying the amount and type of food to be eaten at each meal.

• Encourage her to recognize and verbalize her feelings about her eating behavior. Provide an accepting and nonjudgmental atmosphere, controlling your reactions to her behavior and feelings.

• Encourage the patient to talk about stressful issues, such as achievement, independence, socialization, sexuality, family problems, and control.

• Identify the patient's elimination patterns.

• Assess her suicide potential.

• Refer the patient and her family to the American Anorexia/Bulimia Association and to Anorexia Nervosa and Related Eating Disorders as sources of additional information and support.

• Teach the patient how to keep a food journal to monitor treatment progress.

• Outline the risks of laxative, emetic, and diuretic abuse for the patient.

• Provide assertiveness training to help the patient gain control over her behavior and achieve a realistic and positive self-image.

• If the patient is taking a tricyclic antidepressant, instruct her to take the drug with food. Warn her to avoid consuming alcoholic beverages; exposing herself to sunlight, heat lamps, or tanning beds; and discontinuing the medication without notifying you.

Anorexia nervosa

The key feature of anorexia nervosa is self-imposed starvation resulting from a distorted body image and an intense and irrational fear of gaining weight, even when the patient is obviously emaciated. An anorexic patient is preoccupied with her body size, describes herself as "fat," and commonly expresses dissatisfaction with a particular aspect of her physical appearance. Although the term *anorexia* suggests that the patient's weight loss is associated with a loss of appetite, this is rare. Anorexia nervosa and bulimia nervosa can occur simultaneously. In anorexia nervosa, the refusal to eat may be accompanied by compulsive exercising, self-induced vomiting, or abuse of laxatives or diuretics.

Anorexia occurs in 5% to 10% of the population; about 95% of those affected are women. This disorder occurs primarily in adolescents and young adults but also may affect older women. The occurrence among males is rising. The prognosis varies but improves if the patient is diagnosed early or if she wants to overcome the disorder and seeks help voluntarily. Mortality ranges from 5% to 15%—the highest mortality associated with a psychiatric disturbance. One-third of these deaths can be attributed to suicide.

Causes

No one knows what causes anorexia nervosa. Researchers in neuroendocrinology are seeking a physiologic cause but have found nothing definite. Clearly, social attitudes that equate slimness with beauty play some role in provoking this disorder; family factors also are implicated. Most theorists believe that refusing to eat is a subconscious effort to exert personal control over life.

Signs and symptoms

The patient's history usually reveals a 25% or greater weight loss for no organic reason, coupled with a morbid dread of being fat and a compulsion to be thin. Such a patient tends to be angry and ritualistic. She may report amenorrhea, infertility, loss of libido, fatigue, sleep alterations, intolerance to cold, and constipation.

Hypotension and bradycardia may be present. (See *Complications of anorexia nervosa,* page 144.) Inspection

Complications of anorexia nervosa

Serious medical complications can result from the malnutrition, dehydration, and electrolyte imbalances caused by prolonged starvation, vomiting, or laxative abuse that's typical in anorexia nervosa.

Malnutrition and related problems
For example, malnutrition may cause hypoalbuminemia and subsequent edema or hypokalemia, leading to ventricular arrhythmias and renal failure.

Poor nutrition and dehydration, coupled with laxative abuse, produce changes in the bowel similar to those in chronic inflammatory bowel disease. Frequent vomiting can cause esophageal erosion, ulcers, tears, and bleeding, as well as tooth and gum erosion and dental caries.

Cardiovascular consequences
Cardiovascular complications, which can be life-threatening, include decreased left ventricular muscle mass, chamber size, and myocardial oxygen uptake; reduced cardiac output; hypotension; bradycardia; electrocardiographic changes, such as a nonspecific ST interval, T-wave changes, and a prolonged PR interval; heart failure; and sudden death, possibly caused by ventricular arrhythmias.

Infection and amenorrhea
Anorexia nervosa may increase the patient's susceptibility to infection.

In addition, amenorrhea, which may occur when the patient loses about 25% of her normal body weight, usually is associated with anemia. Possible complications of prolonged amenorrhea include estrogen deficiency (increasing the risk of calcium deficiency and osteoporosis) and infertility. Menses usually return to normal when the patient weighs at least 95% of her normal weight.

---

may reveal an emaciated appearance, with skeletal muscle atrophy, loss of fatty tissue, atrophy of breast tissue, blotchy or sallow skin, lanugo on the face and body, and dryness or loss of scalp hair. Calluses of the knuckles and abrasions and scars on the dorsum of the hand may result from tooth injury during self-induced vomiting. Other signs of vomiting include dental caries and oral or pharyngeal abrasions.

Palpation may disclose painless salivary gland enlargement and bowel distention. Slowed reflexes may occur on percussion. Oddly, the patient usually demonstrates hyperactivity and vigor (despite undernourishment) and may exercise avidly without apparent fatigue.

During psychosocial assessment, the anorexic patient may express a morbid fear of gaining weight and an obsession with her physical appearance. Paradoxically, she also may be obsessed with food, preparing elaborate meals for others. Social regression, including poor sexual adjustment

Diagnosing anorexia nervosa

A diagnosis of anorexia nervosa is made when the patient meets the following criteria put forth in the *DSM-IV:*
• The patient refuses to maintain body weight over a minimal normal weight for age and height (for instance, weight loss leading to maintenance of body weight 15% below that expected); or failure to achieve expected weight gain during a growth period, leading to body weight 15% below that expected.
• The patient experiences intense fear of gaining weight or becoming fat, despite her underweight status.
• The patient has a distorted perception of body weight, size, or shape (that is, the person claims to feel fat even when emaciated or believes that one body area is too fat even when it's obviously underweight).
• In women, absence of at least three consecutive menstrual cycles when otherwise expected to occur.

and fear of failure, is common. Like bulimia nervosa, anorexia nervosa often is associated with depression. The patient may report feelings of despair, hopelessness, and worthlessness as well as suicidal thoughts.

Diagnosis

For characteristic findings in patients with this condition, see *Diagnosing anorexia nervosa.*

In addition, laboratory tests help to identify various disorders and deficiencies and help to rule out endocrine, metabolic, and central nervous system abnormalities; cancer; malabsorption syndrome; and other disorders that cause physical wasting.

Abnormal findings that may accompany a weight loss greater than 30% of normal body weight include:
• low hemoglobin level, platelet count, and white blood cell count
• prolonged bleeding time due to thrombocytopenia
• decreased erythrocyte sedimentation rate
• decreased levels of serum creatinine, blood urea nitrogen, uric acid, cholesterol, total protein, albumin, sodium, potassium, chloride, calcium, and fasting blood glucose (resulting from malnutrition)
• elevated levels of alanine aminotransferase and aspartate aminotransferase in severe starvation states
• elevated serum amylase levels when pancreatitis is not present

• in females, decreased levels of serum luteinizing hormone and follicle-stimulating hormone
• decreased triiodothyronine levels resulting from a lower basal metabolic rate
• dilute urine caused by an impairment in the kidneys' ability to concentrate urine
• nonspecific ST interval, prolonged PR interval, and T-wave changes on the electrocardiogram. Ventricular arrhythmias also may be present.

Treatment

Appropriate treatment aims to promote weight gain or control the patient's compulsive binge eating and purging and to correct malnutrition and the underlying psychological dysfunction. Hospitalization in a medical or psychiatric unit may be required to improve the patient's precarious physical condition. The patient's hospital stay may be as brief as 2 weeks, or his stay may stretch from a few months to 2 years or longer.

A team approach to care often works best. The team provides a combination of aggressive medical management, nutritional counseling, and individual, group, or family psychotherapy or behavior modification therapy. The treatment of anorexia nervosa is difficult and results may be discouraging. Many clinical centers are now developing inpatient and outpatient programs specifically aimed at managing eating disorders.

Treatment for an eating disorder may include behavior modification (privileges depend on weight gain); curtailed activity for physical reasons (such as arrhythmias); vitamin and mineral supplements; a reasonable diet, with or without liquid supplements; subclavian, peripheral, or enteral hyperalimentation (enteral and peripheral routes carry less risk of infection); and group, family, or individual psychotherapy.

All forms of psychotherapy, from psychoanalysis to hypnotherapy, have been used in treating anorexia nervosa, with varying success. To be successful, psychotherapy should address the underlying problems of low self-esteem, guilt, anxiety, feelings of hopelessness and helplessness, and depression.

Special
considerations

• During hospitalization, regularly monitor vital signs, nutritional status, and intake and output. Weigh the patient with an eating disorder daily–before breakfast if possible. Because the patient fears being weighed, vary the weighing routine. Keep in mind that weight should increase from morning to night.

• Help the patient establish a target weight, and support her efforts to achieve this goal.

• Negotiate an adequate food intake with the patient. Be sure that she understands that she'll need to comply with this contract or lose privileges. Frequently offer small portions of food or drinks if the patient wants them. Allow the patient to maintain control over the types and amounts of food eaten, if possible.

• Maintain one-on-one supervision of the patient during meals and for 1 hour afterward to ensure compliance with the dietary treatment program. For the hospitalized anorexic patient, food is considered a medication.

• During an acute anorexic episode, nutritionally complete liquids are more acceptable because they eliminate the need to choose between foods–something the anorexic patient often finds difficult.

• If tube feedings or other special feeding measures become necessary, fully explain these feeding measures to the patient and be ready to discuss her fears or reluctance. Remember to limit the discussion about food itself.

• Anticipate a weight gain of approximately 1 lb (0.5 kg) per week.

• If edema or bloating occurs after the patient has returned to normal eating behavior, reassure her that this phenomenon is temporary. She may fear that she is becoming fat and stop complying with the treatment plan.

• Encourage the patient to recognize and assert her feelings freely. If she understands that she can be assertive, she gradually may learn that expressing her true feelings will not result in her losing control or love.

• If a patient receiving outpatient treatment must be hospitalized, maintain contact with her treatment team to facilitate a smooth return to the outpatient setting.

• Remember that the anorexic patient uses exercise, preoccupation with food, ritualism, manipulation, and lying as mechanisms to preserve the only control she thinks that she has in her life.

• Because the patient and her family may need therapy to uncover and correct dysfunctional patterns, refer them to Anorexia Nervosa and Related Eating Disorders, a national information and support organization. This organization may help them understand what anorexia is, convince them that they need help, and help them find a psychotherapist or medical doctor who is experienced in treating this disorder.

• Teach the patient how to keep a food journal, including the types of food eaten, eating frequency, and feelings associated with eating and exercise.

• Advise family members to avoid discussing food with the patient.

Self-test questions

You can quickly review your comprehension of this chapter on eating disorders by answering the following questions. The correct answers to these questions and their rationales appear on pages 165 and 166.

Case history questions

Barbara Binns, a 31-year-old divorcee, is a hostess in a fine restaurant. Recently, she admitted to behaviors that meet the criteria for bulimia nervosa: She eats huge portions of food when by herself and then feels guilty about the amount she has consumed. She has been using laxatives and enemas, and she can make herself vomit. Since her divorce two years ago, Barbara has doubled the number of aerobics classes she takes each week.

1. Barbara was able to keep her eating disorder hidden for many years because she:
    a. was perceived by her friends as a perfect career woman.
    b. maintained her weight within normal range.
    c. talked as if good nutrition was important to her.
    d. had a seemingly happy social life.

2. Barbara's frequent secret eating binges were followed by feelings of:
   a. anger.
   b. depression.
   c. unreality.
   d. humiliation.

3. Preferred foods for Barbara's binge eating were most likely:
   a. high in fat.
   b. chewy and flavorful.
   c. sweet and high in carbohydrates.
   d. soft and high in bulk.

4. Barbara initially controlled her weight with exercise, but soon resorted to vomiting and purging. Although she did not appear ill, an examination revealed:
   a. cardiac failure.
   b. an esophageal tear.
   c. severe dehydration.
   d. electrolyte imbalances.

Amelia Hibert was diagnosed with anorexia nervosa at age 19. She vigorously exercised two to three times a day. While she often prepared elaborate meals for her family, she would always insist that she was "too full" to eat more than a salad.

5. Amelia demonstrated the key feature of anorexia, which is:
   a. self-imposed starvation.
   b. a distorted body image.
   c. an irrational fear of gaining weight.
   d. dissatisfaction with the appearance of her hips and thighs.

6. Amelia's weight loss, which was typical for an anorexic patient, was found to be:
   a. 10%.
   b. 15%.
   c. 20%.
   d. 25%.

7. With this degree of weight loss, Amelia experienced the associated dysfunction of:
  a. osteoporosis.
  b. chronic inflammatory bowel disease.
  c. amenorrhea.
  d. excessive fatigue.

8. Amelia responded well to an outpatient treatment using behavior modification, nutritional counseling, and psychotherapy. She achieved the desired weekly weight gain of:
  a. ½ lb (0.2 kg).
  b. 1 lb (0.5 kg).
  c. 2 lbs (0.9 kg).
  d. 3 lbs (1.4 kg).

Selected References
and Self-Test Answers and Rationales

Selected References

Anguilera, D.C. *Crisis Intervention: Theory and Methodology,* 7th ed. St. Louis: Mosby–Year Book, Inc., 1994.

Barry, P.D. *Mental Health and Mental Illness,* 5th ed. Philadelphia: J.B. Lippincott Co., 1994.

Bruno, Frank J. *Psychological Symptoms.* New York: John Wiley & Sons, 1994.

Diagnostic and Statistical Manual of Mental Disorders, 4th ed. Washington, D.C.: American Psychiatric Association, 1994.

Goldberg, T.E., et al. "Contrasts between Patients with Affective Disorders and Patients with Schizophrenia on a Neuropsychological Test Battery," *American Journal of Psychiatry* 150(9):1355-62, September 1993.

Isselbacher, K., et al., eds. *Harrison's Principles of Internal Medicine,* 13th ed. New York: McGraw-Hill Book Co., 1994.

Jensen, P.S., et al. "Anxiety and Depressive Disorders in Attention Deficit Disorder with Hyperactivity: New Findings," *American Journal of Psychiatry* 150(8):1203-09, August 1993.

Physician's Drug Handbook, 6th ed. Springhouse, Pa.: Springhouse Corp., 1995.

Professional Handbook of Diagnostic Tests. Springhouse, Pa.: Springhouse Corp., 1995.

Shueman, S., et al., eds. *Managed Behavioral Health Care: An Industry Perspective.* Springfield, Ill.: Charles C. Thomas Publishing Co., 1994.

Stuart, G.W., and Sundeen, S.J. *Principles and Practice of Psychiatric Nursing,* 5th ed. St. Louis: Mosby–Year Book, Inc., 1994.

Townsend, M.C. *Psychiatric/Mental Health Nursing: Concepts of Care.* Philadelphia: F.A. Davis, 1993.

Waddington, J.L. "Schizophrenia: Developmental Neuroscience and Pathobiology," *Lancet* 341(8844):531-36, February 27, 1993.

Self-Test Answers and Rationales

Chapter 1:
Introduction

1. d Isolation, fear of violent crimes, and loneliness have contributed to a rise in depression among elderly people. Combat veterans, rape victims, and child abuse victims struggle to cope with trauma they've experienced. The loss of support systems can strain anyone's ability to cope with even minor problems. When an individual sees himself as ineffective in usual roles, self-esteem falters.

2. d Axis V measures how well the patient has functioned over the past year, and encompasses the patient's current level of functioning. Axis II speaks to personality disorders and mental retardation, Axis III to general medical conditions, and Axis IV documents the effect of psychosocial and environmental stressors on the patient.

3. b Patients experiencing socioeconomic hardships are more likely to show distress during an illness. Also, such information may provide clues to the patient's current problem. Demographic data establishes a baseline and validates the patient's record. Cultural and religious beliefs and values affect a patient's response to illness and his adaptation to care. Cultural background and personal values influence a patient's answers to hypothetical questions.

4. c Evaluate the patient's mood by asking him to describe his current feelings. How the patient responds to the interviewer is part of behavior assessment. Evaluating his orientation to time, place, and person assesses thought processes and cognitive function. Questioning his understanding of the significance of his illness assesses the patient's degree of insight.

5. a The Cognitive Assessment Scale measures orientation, general knowledge, mental ability, and psychomotor function. The Cognitive Capacity Screening Examination measures orientation, memory, calculation, and language. The Global Deterioration Scale assesses and stages primary degenerative dementia, based on orientation, memory, and neurologic function. The Functional Dementia Scale measures orientation, affect, and the ability to perform activities of daily living.

6. a An EEG graphically records the brain's electrical activity. Abnormal results may indicate organic disease, psychotropic drug use, or certain psychological disorders. A computed tomography (CT) scan can help detect brain contusions or calcifications, cerebral atrophy, hydrocephalus, inflammation, space-occupying lesions, and vascular abnormalities. A magnetic resonance imaging scan provides superior contrast of soft tissues and sharper differentiation of normal and abnormal tissues, as compared to conventional X-rays and CT scans. A positron emission topography scan is used mainly for diagnosing neuropsychiatric problems and some mental illnesses.

Chapter 2: Disorders of Infancy, Childhood, and Adolescence

1. b The recognized levels for moderate mental retardation are IQ of 35-40 to 50-55. The other recognized levels of mental retardation are as follows: mild retardation, IQ of 50-55 to approximately 70; severe retardation, IQ of 20-25 to 35-40; and profound retardation, IQ of less than 20-25.

2. d A primary goal of mental retardation treatment is to develop the patient's strengths as fully as possible. Special education and training are necessary to help achieve the goals. Special considerations in treatment include promoting continuity of care for a hospitalized patient with mental retardation by acting as a liaison for parents and other health care professionals involved in his care, and suggesting ways for parents to cope with the guilt, frustration, and exhaustion that often accompany caring for a severely retarded child.

3. c In Tourette syndrome, tics occur many times a day (usually in bouts) nearly every day, or intermittently for more than a year. Tics that have occurred for at least 4 weeks but no longer than 12 consecutive months help to define transient tic disorder. Single or multiple motor or vocal tics, but not both, are present at some time during chronic motor or vocal tic disorder. In all tics, the disturbance causes marked distress or significant impairment in social, occupational, or other important areas of functioning.

4. d Haloperidol is the drug of choice for Tourette syndrome. Pimozide and clonidine are alternative choices for patients who can't tolerate or don't respond well to haloperidol. Antianxiety agents may be useful in dealing with secondary anxiety but do not reduce the severity or frequency of the tics.

5. a Marked impairment in the use of nonverbal behaviors such as eye-to-eye gaze, facial expression, body postures, and gestures to regulate social interactions is a characteristic defining qualitative impairment in social interaction. Qualitative impairment in communication encompasses characteristics such as delay in, or total lack of, the development of spoken language. Restrictive repetitive and stereotyped patterns in behavior, interests, and activities are manifested by such characteristics as stereotyped and repetitive motor mannerisms or persistent preoccupation with parts of objects. Diagnosis of autism also encompasses delays or abnormal functioning in at least one of the following areas, with onset prior to age three: social interaction; language as used in social communication; or symbolic or imaginative play.

6. c To reduce self-destructive behaviors, first physically stop the child from harming himself, while firmly saying "no." When he responds to your voice, first give a primary reward (such as food); later, substitute verbal or physical reinforcement (such as "good," or a hug or pat on the back). Providing pleasurable sensory and motor stimulation, which encourages appropriate behavior and helps eliminate inappropriate behavior, is one of the behavioral techniques used to reduce symptoms and increase the child's ability to respond.

7. d For a younger child, the disorder will be most evident in his inability to wait in line, remain seated, wait his turn, and concentrate on one activity until it is completed. An older child or adult will be impulsive, emotionally labile, easily distracted, inattentive, and disorganized; have trouble keeping track of tools and materials; hand in work late; daydream; and be easily distracted by irrelevant thoughts, sounds, or sights.

8. d Some individuals will benefit from medication. It is important to identify the particular symptoms you want to decrease and track them carefully to determine the effectiveness of the medication. These symptoms may include any of the diagnostic criteria characteristic of inattention, hyperactivity, or impulsivity as identified in this child.

Chapter 3: Psychoactive Substance Abuse (Alcoholism and Drug Abuse)

1. a One characteristic of substance intoxication is the development of a reversible substance-specific syndrome due to recent ingestion of, or exposure to, a substance. Continued substance use despite having persistent or recurrent social or interpersonal problems caused or exacerbated by the effects of the substance is a characteristic of substance abuse. In substance dependence, a great deal of time is spent in activities necessary to obtain the substance, use the substance, or recover from its effects. The need for increased amounts of the substance to achieve the desired effect (or to achieve intoxication) is a characteristic of tolerance.

2. c An offspring of one alcoholic parent is seven to eight times more likely to become an alcoholic than is a peer without such a parent. Numerous biological, psychological and sociocultural factors have been implicated, with biological factors including genetic or biochemical abnormalities, nutritional deficiencies, endocrine imbalances, and allergic responses. None of the other distractors are correct.

3. d Assessing for alcoholism may be difficult because people with alcohol dependence may hide or deny their addiction and may temporarily manage to maintain a functional life. Blackouts, violence, and untreated, unexplained injuries are only a few of many assessment criteria for alcoholism. They may be absent, and the patient's alcoholism defined by other characteristics.

4. c After abstinence or reduction of alcohol intake, manifestations of withdrawal may vary, beginning shortly after drinking has stopped and lasting for 5 to 7 days. The patient initially experiences anorexia, nausea, anxiety, fever, insomnia, diaphoresis, and tremor, progressing to severe tremulousness, agitation, and possibly, hallucinations and violent

behavior. Major motor seizures, also known as "rum fits," can occur during withdrawal.

5. c A blood alcohol level of 0.10% weight volume (200 mg/dl) is accepted as the level of intoxication. Levels of 0.05% and 0.075% would not qualify as intoxication, while a level of 0.20% would be double the required intoxication level.

6. b Aversion therapy uses a daily oral dose of disulfiram to prevent compulsive drinking. Diazepam is a benzodiazepine tranquilizer used to relieve overwhelming anxiety during rehabilitation. Prochlorperazine, a piperazine phenothiazine antipsychotic also may be used for short-term treatment of moderate anxiety. Promazine, an aliphatic phenothiazine, may be used to control hyperactivity and psychosis.

7. d Constricted pupils occur with opiate use or withdrawal; dilated pupils, with the use of hallucinogens or amphetamines. Perforation of the nasal septum mucosa occurs with prolonged use of cocaine (drug sniffing). Central nervous system (CNS) stimulants and some hallucinogens precipitate acute-onset hypertension and cardiac arrhythmias.

8. b To minimize the severe physical discomfort of opioid withdrawal, chronic opioid abusers commonly are detoxified with methadone, a pharmacologically similar drug. Naloxone may be prescribed to reverse severe CNS effects. An anticholinergic would be prescribed to relieve GI distress. Antianxiety agents may be administered temporarily, but are prescribed more specifically for the severe agitation experienced by cocaine abusers.

Chapter 4:
Schizophrenic
Disorders

1. b The *DSM-IV* criteria for schizophrenia states that two or more of the characteristic symptoms must have been present for a significant portion of time during a 1-month period (less if successfully treated). Only one criterion symptom is required if delusions are bizarre or hallucinations consist of a voice keeping up a running commentary on the person's behavior or thoughts, or two or more voices conversing with each other. Diagnosis does not require 3 or 4 or more symptoms to be present.

2. c Echopraxia is involuntary repetition of movements observed in others. Echolalia is meaningless repetition of words or phrases; clang associations, use of words that rhyme or sound alike in an illogical or nonsensical manner; word salad, illogical word groupings.

3. d The belief that one's thought or wishes can control other people or events is magical thinking. An illusion is a false sensory perception with some basis in reality. A delusion is a false idea or belief accepted as real by the patient. Ambivalence is the coexistence of strong negative and positive feelings.

4. a In schizophrenia, hallucinations (false sensory perceptions with no basis in reality) are usually visual or auditory. However, they also may occasionally be olfactory (smell), gustatory (taste), or tactile (touch).

5. a Antipsychotic or neuroleptic drugs appear to work by blocking postsynaptic dopamine receptors. Given the biological hypothesis that schizophrenia results from excessive activity at dopaminergic synapses, such drugs have been the primary treatment for schizophrenia for more than 30 years. Dopaminergic drugs stimulate production and release of dopamine and would not be prescribed. Other psychiatric drugs, such as antidepressants and anxiolytics, may also be prescribed to control associated symptoms.

6. d Certain medical conditions exaggerate the risk of delusional disorders: head injury, chronic alcoholism, deafness and aging. Delusional disorders commonly begin in middle or late adulthood, but can occur at any age. Schizophrenia more commonly begins in adolescence or early adulthood, and can also occur in childhood. The incidence of delusional disorders and of schizophrenia is about equal in men and women.

7. c Routine blood monitoring is essential to detect the estimated 1% to 2% of all patients taking clozapine who develop agranulocytosis, a potentially fatal blood disorder characterized by a low white blood cell count and pronounced neutropenia. Thrombocytopenia (low platelet count) and anemias (aplastic, absent, or low red blood cell [RBC] production; hemolytic, excessive RBC destruction) do not occur relative to this drug therapy.

Chapter 5:
Mood
Disorders

1. c The *DSM-IV* criteria for a bipolar II disorder state that there has never been a manic episode or a mixed episode. One or more major depressive episodes have occurred, along with at least one hypomanic episode. Both bipolar I and bipolar II criteria speak to the occurrence of significant functional impairment (social, occupational, or other).

2. b In cyclothymia, a variant of bipolar disorders, numerous episodes of hypomania and depressive symptoms are too mild to meet the criteria for bipolar illnesses or major depression. In some patients, bipolar disorders assume a seasonal pattern, characterized by a cyclic relationship between the onset of a mood episode and a particular 60-day period of the year. Mixed episodes occur in bipolar I disorder but not in bipolar II disorder. Mood disorders are so classified because they meet the *DSM-IV* criteria and are not better accounted for by a schizoaffective disorder and are not superimposed on a schizophrenic disorder.

3. b Widely used in the treatment of bipolar I disorder, lithium proves highly effective in relieving and preventing manic episodes, and may prevent recurrence of depressive episodes. Carbamazepine, a potent antimanic, often is effective in lithium-resistant patients. Valproic acid and clonazepam may be used to treat mood disorders either alone or along with lithium.

4. d Suicide is the most serious complication of major depression, resulting when the patient's feelings of worthlessness, guilt, and hopelessness are so overwhelming that he no longer considers life worth living. Major depression also can alter social, family, and occupational functioning.

5. d The multiple causes of depression are not completely understood. Current research suggests possible genetic, familial, biochemical, physical, psychological, and social causes, but does not zero in on any one of these as *the* cause.

6. c At least five symptoms must have been present during the same two-week period nearly every day and represent a change from previous functioning. One of these symptoms must be either depressed mood or loss of interest in previously pleasurable activities. The other symptoms noted may or may not have been experienced, as long as at least five out of nine listed in the *DSM-IV* occurred.

7. b Selective serotonin reuptake inhibitors (SSRIs) such as fluoxetine are increasingly the drugs of first choice in depression because they are effective and have fewer disturbing adverse effects. Monoamine oxidase inhibitors require dietary modifications, but may be used for patients who do not respond well to tricyclic antidepressants or SSRIs. All antidepressive drug therapy aims at preventing recurrent depression, but this outcome cannot be guaranteed on any one regimen.

8. d Six to 12 electroconvulsive therapy treatments usually are required to treat depression, although improvement may be evident after only a few treatments.

**Chapter 6:
Anxiety
Disorders**

1. c Specific phobias such as acrophobia usually begin in childhood. The onset of a social phobia is apt to occur in late childhood or early adolescence; thus, phobias usually are in place before adulthood, although symptoms are apt to increase over time. Most phobic patients have no family history of psychiatric illness, including phobias.

2. d A patient who routinely avoids the object of his phobia may report a loss of self-esteem and feelings of weakness, cowardice, or ineffectiveness. He may also exhibit signs of mild depression because he has not mastered the phobia, as opposed to increased anxiety. Avoidance no longer suffices to make him feel comfortable or even relieved; otherwise, he would not have sought help in dealing with it.

3. b The goal of treatment is to help the patient function effectively. Systematic desensitization, a behavioral therapy, may be more effective than drugs, especially if it includes encouragement, instruction, and suggestion. Psychotherapy may be helpful; however, the patient should not be forced to gain insight, as this may aggravate anxiety. Antianxiety agents may temporarily help to relieve symptoms, as may antidepressants in agoraphobia (fear of being alone or in open spaces).

4. d The patient with panic disorder is at high risk for a psychoactive substance use disorder, resorting to alcohol or anxiolytics in an attempt to relieve fear. By their very nature, panic attacks involve intense anxiety, with further anxiety generated by worry between attacks about when the next one will occur. Panic disorder does not involve depression, and it is depression that most often triggers the risk for suicide.

5. a If left alone during a panic attack, the patient may become even more anxious, so stay with her until the attack subsides, maintaining a calm and serene approach indicating your control of the situation. Don't resort to loud speech as the unnecessary stimulus may overwhelm her, and don't offer unrealistic reassurance. Avoid touching the patient until rapport is established, as touch may not be reassuring to a stimulated and frightened individual. Also don't hold her still, but allow her to pace about to expend excess energy. The patient will be unable to focus on complex instructions or activities, so provide one direction at a time in short, simple sentences.

6. d Performing a compulsive behavior reduces the patient's anxiety, but reinforces the probability that the behavior will recur. The compulsion is a ritualistic, repetitive, and involuntary defense behavior. Patients with obsessive-compulsive disorder are prone to abuse psychoactive substances, such as alcohol and anxiolytics, in an attempt to relieve their anxiety.

7. d Support groups are highly effective in treatment of posttraumatic stress syndrome, providing a forum in which victims of this disorder can work through their feelings with others who have had similar conflicts. These individuals may also benefit from relaxation therapy, progressive desensitization, or psychotherapy, but such treatments would be conducted outside of the support group.

8. c Theorists share a common premise about the cause of generalized anxiety disorder: conflict, whether intrapsychic, sociopersonal, or interpersonal, promotes an anxiety state. Thus anxiety is a reaction to an internal threat, while fear is a reaction to danger from a particular external source. Posttraumatic stress disorder occurs in response to an extremely distressing event. A brain lesion is one cause postulated for obsessive-compulsive disorder.

Chapter 7: Somatoform Disorders

1. b Ongoing assessment should focus on new signs and symptoms and any change in old ones to avoid missing a developing physical disease. Mrs. Novak should not have been diagnosed as having a somatization disorder until investigation indicated that no known medical condition could fully explain her symptoms. Investigating her anxiety or depression will be useful only if it helps her to live with her signs and symptoms, not in an effort to discount her symptoms. Patients with somatization disorder are not making up their symptoms. Rather, these are involuntary and the patient truly wishes to feel better.

2. d The most important aspect of treatment is a continuing supportive relationship with a care provider who acknowledges the patient's signs and symptoms and is willing to help her live with them. The patient with somatization disorder seldom acknowledges any psychological aspect of her illness and rejects psychiatric treatment. The ongoing supportive relationship may have a secondary effect of reducing this patient's anxiety, but that is not to say that her symptoms will be relieved.

3. a The loss of physical function in conversion reaction is involuntary, allowing a patient to resolve a psychological conflict through the loss of a specific physical function. A voluntary loss would be considered factitious or malingering.

4. c It is important to help the patient maintain integrity of the affected system. In Rev. Ralphson's case, a speech therapist could prescribe exercises to prevent loss of vocal muscle capabilities. Don't injure your therapeutic relationship with this patient by asking or insisting that he speak, placing him in situations where speech is requisite, or repeatedly reminding him that no physical cause exists. Psychotherapy, relaxation therapy, hypnosis, or other therapies should help him to deal with the triggering psychological cause, so that he would again be able to use his voice, perhaps beginning with a different form such as singing.

5. d Regularly scheduled analgesic doses can be more effective than administering analgesic medication on an "as needed" (p.r.n.) basis, which forces unneeded confrontations and can increase anxiety. The patient should be told clearly which medication is being used to avoid having him feel that his pain is not being taken seriously. The use of placebos may indeed relieve pain if the patient responds to the drug by releasing endorphins; thus, their use does not determine the presence or absence of pain. All pain is real to the individual experiencing it.

6. c Stress increases the risk of developing hypochondriasis. It can begin at any age, but onset most frequently occurs between ages 20 and 30, so aging is not a factor. Hypochondriasis appears to be equally common in men and women. It is not due to other mental disorders, such as schizophrenia, mood disorder, or somatization disorder.

7. b The patient with hypochondriasis is unaware of having unmet needs and does not consciously develop the reported symptoms. Thus, the patient does not knowingly assume a sick role to ensure that particular needs are met, although this is usually the outcome. Hypochondriasis is not a circumscribed concern about appearance (as in body dysmorphic disorder).

8. d When caring for a hypochondriacal patient, recognize that the patient will never be symptom-free. You may reduce her symptoms over time by helping her to develop more effective coping strategies, but you cannot eliminate them. Don't challenge the patient's symptoms or try to force her to give up her disease, as this can simply drive the patient away to yet another medical evaluation.

1. a A complex disturbance of identity and memory, dissociative identity disorder (formerly referred to as "multiple personality disorder") is characterized by the existence of two or more distinct, fully integrated personalities in the same person. Wandering or traveling while assuming a different personality and later not recalling what happened is characteristic of dissociative fugue. In dissociative amnesia, there is sudden inability to recall important personal information that cannot be explained by ordinary forgetfulness. This patient typically is unable to recall all events that occurred during a specific time period, but other types of recall disturbances also are possible.

2. a Usually, one personality is unaware of the other; thus, Ashley would assume that these clothes belong to someone else. Buying clothes of this type, even to give them away, would be inconsistent with her usual personality, as she would not approve of them or associate with anyone who would wear such clothes. Paranoia is not a part of this disorder, so she would not assume that they were in her closet to be used against her.

3. b Psychotherapy is essential to unite the personalities and prevent the personality from splitting again. Behavior modification would not be appropriate, as it is not the behavior of the second personality that must be addressed, but the personality itself. Drug therapy might be used supportively as an adjunct to psychotherapy, but not as a substitute.

4. a Although the fugue state usually is brief (hours to days) it can last for many months and carry the patient far from home.

5. d Dissociative fugue typically follows an extremely stressful event, such as combat experience, a natural disaster, a violent or abusive confrontation, or personal rejection. Heavy alcohol use may be a predisposing factor, but not a family disagreement, intermittent bouts of depression, or a long period of general unhappiness.

6. c Dissociative amnesia commonly occurs during war and natural disasters. It follows severe psychological stress, often involving a *threat* of physical injury or death. Heavy alcohol use and psychotropic drug use are not causes of this disorder.

7. b The patient with depersonalization disorder may complain of feeling detached from her entire being and body, as if watching herself from a distance or living in a dream. She also may report sensory anesthesia, a loss of self-control, difficulty speaking, and feelings of derealization and loss of reality.

8. a Common findings during the assessment interview include symptoms of depression, obsessive rumination, physical complaints, anxiety, fear of going insane, a disturbed sense of time (but not place), and a prolonged recall time (but not inability to recall personal history details).

Chapter 9: Eating Disorders

1. b Typically, bulimic patients maintain their weight within normal range, although it may fluctuate. Thus, unlike the anorexic patient, the bulimic usually can keep her eating disorder hidden. While bulimics commonly are perceived by others as "perfect," nonbulimic individuals may also be awarded this label. Demonstrating surface happiness among her social set and talking about the importance of good nutrition also are not specific to this diagnosis, although they could be used to "cover" for her bulimic behaviors.

2. d The essential features of bulimia include eating binges followed by feelings of guilt, humiliation, and self-deprecation. Bulimia also may be associated with depression. Anger is not a feature; indeed, bulimic patients have difficulty expressing anger. Feelings of unreality are part of depersonalization disorder.

3. c The preferred food for binge eating is usually sweet, soft, and high in calories and carbohydrates, rather than chewy and flavorful or high in bulk. Fats contribute to the high caloric content but are not the primary feature.

4. d Electrolyte imbalances such as metabolic alkalosis, hypochloremia, and hypokalemia occur in bulimia when vomiting and purging and diuretics are used to control weight.

Dehydration also can occur, but if severe, the patient would look ill, as she would with cardiac failure (usually related to ipecac syrup intoxication) and definitely with the rare complication of an esophageal tear.

5. a The key feature of anorexia nervosa is self-imposed starvation. This results from a distorted body image and an intense and irrational fear of gaining weight. The individual describes herself as fat and often is dissatisfied with a particular aspect of her physical appearance (such as her hips and thighs).

6. d Weight loss in anorexia nervosa usually is 25% or greater for no organic reason. However, weight loss leading to maintenance of body weight 15% below that desired for age and height is part of the *DSM-IV* diagnostic criteria. Lesser percentages of loss with no organic reason would, of course, also be a concern if they placed the individual below normal weight ranges for her height, age, and other nutritional assessment criteria.

7. c Amenorrhea may occur when the patient loses about 25% of her normal body weight. This can lead to associated estrogen deficiency problems such as osteoporosis. Bowel inflammation is associated with laxative abuse in addition to poor nutrition and dehydration, and Amelia did not use laxatives at this point in her illness. Oddly, the patient usually demonstrates restless activity and vigor (despite her undernourishment) and may exercise avidly without apparent fatigue.

8. b With appropriate supervised food intake, the anorexic patient should gain about 1 lb (0.5 kg) per week. Less gain would be reason to renegotiate food intake with the patient. Greater gains might be more indicative of fluid retention than actual tissue gain.

Appendices and Index

Recommended Laboratory Tests During Psychotropic Drug Therapy

Long-term psychotropic drug therapy can cause physiologic abnormalities best detected by laboratory tests. The following chart lists tests that should be performed for patients taking antidepressants, antimanics, antipsychotics, anxiolytics, and sedative-hypnotics. The drugs appear in alphabetical order according to primary therapeutic use. Laboratory tests also appear in alphabetical order.

DRUG	TESTS	PURPOSE	SPECIAL CONSIDERATIONS
Antidepressants			
Amitriptyline	Blood counts	To detect blood dyscrasias	Establish baseline and repeat periodically, especially in symptomatic patients.
	Electrocardiogram (ECG)	To detect cardiotoxicity	Establish baseline and repeat periodically, especially in patients receiving high doses.
	Liver function tests	To detect hepatotoxicity	Establish baseline and repeat periodically; asymptomatic elevations of transaminase and alkaline phosphatase levels, which can progress to signs of hepatic failure, have occurred in patients receiving tricyclic antidepressants (TCAs).
	Ophthalmologic exams, including tonometry	To detect glaucoma	Anticholinergic effects may exacerbate glaucoma.
Amoxapine	Blood counts	To detect blood dyscrasias	Establish baseline and repeat periodically, especially in symptomatic patients.
	ECG	To detect cardiotoxicity	Establish baseline and repeat periodically, especially in patients receiving high doses.
	Liver function tests	To detect hepatotoxicity	Establish baseline and repeat periodically; asymptomatic elevations of transaminase and alkaline phosphatase levels, which can progress to signs of hepatic failure, have occurred in patients receiving TCAs.
	Ophthalmologic exams, including tonometry	To detect glaucoma	Anticholinergic effects may exacerbate glaucoma.

DRUG	TESTS	PURPOSE	SPECIAL CONSIDERATIONS
Antidepressants *(continued)*			
Bupropion	Blood counts	To detect blood dyscrasias	Establish baseline and repeat periodically, especially in symptomatic patients.
	ECG	To detect cardiotoxicity	Establish baseline and repeat periodically; bupropion has minimal effects on ECG.
	Body weight	To detect excessive weight loss	Anorectic action noted with short-term use.
Clomipramine	Blood counts	To detect blood dyscrasias	Establish baseline and repeat periodically, especially in symptomatic patients.
	ECG	To detect cardiotoxicity	Establish baseline and repeat periodically, especially in patients receiving high doses.
	Liver function tests	To detect hepatotoxicity	Establish baseline and repeat periodically; asymptomatic elevations of transaminase and alkaline phosphatase levels, which can progress to signs of hepatic failure, have occurred in patients receiving TCAs.
	Ophthalmologic exams, including tonometry	To detect glaucoma	Anticholinergic effects may exacerbate glaucoma.
Desipramine	Blood counts	To detect blood dyscrasias	Establish baseline and repeat periodically, especially in symptomatic patients.
	ECG	To detect cardiotoxicity	Establish baseline and repeat periodically, especially in patients receiving high doses.
	Liver function	To detect hepatotoxicity	Establish baseline and repeat periodically; asymptomatic elevations of transaminase and alkaline phosphatase levels, which can progress to signs of hepatic failure, have occurred in patients receiving TCAs.
	Ophthalmologic exams, including tonometry	To detect glaucoma	Anticholinergic effects may exacerbate glaucoma.

(continued)

DRUG	TESTS	PURPOSE	SPECIAL CONSIDERATIONS
Antidepressants *(continued)*			
Doxepine	Blood counts	To detect blood dyscrasias	Establish baseline and repeat periodically, especially in symptomatic patients.
	ECG	To detect cardiotoxicity	Establish baseline and repeat periodically, especially in patients receiving high doses.
	Liver function tests	To detect hepatotoxicity	Establish baseline and repeat periodically; asymptomatic elevations of transaminase and alkaline phosphatase levels, which can progress to signs of hepatic failure, have occurred in patients receiving TCAs.
	Ophthalmologic exams, including tonometry	To detect glaucoma	Anticholinergic effects may exacerbate glaucoma.
Fluoxetine	Blood counts	To detect blood dyscrasias	Establish baseline and repeat periodically, especially in symptomatic patients.
	Body weight	To detect excessive weight loss	Anorectic action noted with short-term use.
	ECG	To detect cardiotoxicity	Establish baseline and repeat periodically; fluoxetine has minimal effects on ECG.
	Ophthalmologic exams, including tonometry	To detect glaucoma	Anticholinergic effects may exacerbate glaucoma.
Imipramine	Blood counts	To detect blood dyscrasias	Establish baseline and repeat periodically, especially in symptomatic patients.
	ECG	To detect cardiotoxicity	Establish baseline and repeat periodically, especially in patients receiving high doses.
	Liver function tests	To detect hepatotoxicity	Establish baseline and repeat periodically; asymptomatic elevations of transaminase and alkaline phosphatase levels, which can progress to signs of hepatic failure, have occurred in patients receiving TCAs.
	Ophthalmologic exams, including tonometry	To detect glaucoma	Anticholinergic effects may exacerbate glaucoma.

DRUG	TESTS	PURPOSE	SPECIAL CONSIDERATIONS
Antidepressants *(continued)*			
Isocarboxazid	Blood counts	To detect blood dyscrasias	Establish baseline and repeat periodically; normocytic and normochromic anemia, leukocytosis, agranulocytosis, and thrombocytopenia have occurred with monoamine oxidase (MAO) inhibitors.
	Blood pressure	To detect toxicity	May cause orthostatic hypotension, especially in hypertensive patients.
	Liver function studies	To detect hepatotoxicity	Prevalent in patients on prolonged, high-dose therapy.
	Ophthalmologic exams	To detect toxicity	Prolonged use rarely leads to amblyopia, visual disturbances, or glaucoma.
Maprotiline	Blood counts	To detect blood dyscrasias	Establish baseline and repeat periodically, especially in symptomatic patients.
	ECG	To detect cardiotoxicity	Establish baseline and repeat periodically, especially in patients receiving high doses.
	Liver function tests	To detect hepatotoxicity	Establish baseline and repeat periodically; asymptomatic elevations of transaminase and alkaline phosphatase levels, which can progress to signs of hepatic failure, have occurred in patients receiving TCAs.
	Ophthalmologic exams, including tonometry	To detect glaucoma	Anticholinergic effects may exacerbate glaucoma.
Nortriptyline	Blood counts	To detect blood dyscrasias	Establish baseline and repeat periodically, especially in symptomatic patients.
	ECG	To detect cardiotoxicity	Establish baseline and repeat periodically, especially in patients receiving high doses.
	Liver function tests	To detect hepatotoxicity	Establish baseline and repeat periodically; asymptomatic elevations of transaminase and alkaline phosphatase levels, which can progress to signs of hepatic failure, have occurred in patients receiving TCAs.
	Ophthalmologic exams, including tonometry	To detect glaucoma	Anticholinergic effects may exacerbate glaucoma.

(continued)

DRUG	TESTS	PURPOSE	SPECIAL CONSIDERATIONS
Antidepressants *(continued)*			
Paroxetine	Body weight assessment	To detect weight gain	Weight gain is a prevalent adverse effect.
	Electrolyte panel	To measure sodium levels	Low sodium levels have been reported.
Phenelzine	Blood counts	To detect blood dyscrasias	Establish baseline and repeat periodically; normocytic and normochromic anemia, leukocytosis, agranulocytosis, and thrombocytopenia have been reported with MAO inhibitors.
	Blood pressure	To detect toxicity	May cause orthostatic hypotension, especially in hypertensive patients.
	Liver function studies	To detect hepatotoxicity	Prevalent in patients on prolonged, high-dose therapy.
	Ophthalmologic exams	To detect toxicity	Prolonged use may be associated rarely with amblyopia, visual disturbances, or glaucoma.
Protriptyline	Blood counts	To detect blood dyscrasias	Establish baseline and repeat periodically, especially in symptomatic patients.
	ECG	To detect cardiotoxicity	Establish baseline and repeat periodically, especially in patients receiving high doses.
	Liver function tests	To detect hepatotoxicity	Establish baseline and repeat periodically; asymptomatic elevations of transaminase and alkaline phosphatase levels, which can progress to signs of hepatic failure, have occurred in patients receiving TCAs.
	Ophthalmologic exams, including tonometry	To detect glaucoma	Anticholinergic effects may exacerbate glaucoma.
Sertraline	ECG	To detect arrhythmias	Palpitations and tachycardia may occur.
	Ophthalmologic examination	To detect visual abnormalities	Conjunctivitis and abnormal vision and accommodation may occur.

DRUG	TESTS	PURPOSE	SPECIAL CONSIDERATIONS
Antidepressants *(continued)*			
Tranylcypro-mine	Blood counts	To detect blood dyscrasias	Establish baseline and repeat periodically; normocytic and normochromic anemia, leukocytosis, agranulocytosis, and thrombocytopenia have been reported with MAO inhibitors.
	Blood pressure	To detect toxicity	May cause orthostatic hypotension, especially in hypertensive patients.
	Liver function studies	To detect hepatotoxicity	Hepatotoxicity is prevalent with prolonged, high-dose therapy.
	Ophthalmologic exams	To detect toxicity	Prolonged use may be associated rarely with amblyopia, visual disturbances, or glaucoma.
Trazodone	Blood counts	To detect blood dyscrasias	Establish baseline and repeat periodically, especially in symptomatic patients.
	ECG	To detect cardiotoxicity	Establish baseline and repeat periodically, especially in patients receiving high doses.
Trimipramine	Blood counts	To detect blood dyscrasias	Establish baseline and check periodically, especially in symptomatic patients.
	ECG	To detect cardiotoxicity	Establish baseline and repeat periodically, especially in patients receiving high doses.
	Liver function tests	To detect hepatotoxicity	Establish baseline and repeat periodically; asymptomatic elevations of transaminase and alkaline phosphatase levels, which can progress to signs of hepatic failure, have occurred in patients receiving TCAs.
	Ophthalmologic exams, including tonometry	To detect glaucoma	Anticholinergic effects may exacerbate glaucoma.
Venlafaxine	ECG	To detect change in heart rate	Increases in number of beats per minute have been reported.
	Serum cholesterol	To detect increase in cholesterol	Increases (by about 3%) of cholesterol have been reported.
	Thyroid function tests	To measure thyroid levels	Increases and decreases have occurred.

(continued)

DRUG	TESTS	PURPOSE	SPECIAL CONSIDERATIONS
Antimanic agent			
Lithium	Blood counts	To detect blood dyscrasias	Establish baseline and repeat periodically.
	Renal function tests	To detect nephron atrophy	Establish baseline renal function (serum creatinine, urinalysis) every 1 to 2 months for the first 6 months, then every 6 months thereafter.
	Serum electrolytes (particularly sodium)	To prevent toxicity	Sodium depletion can decrease lithium clearance and increase risk of toxicity. Patients should be advised to use sodium (salt) liberally.
	Serum lithium levels	To prevent toxicity	Toxic effects associated with levels above 1.5 mEq/liter.
	Thyroid function studies	To evaluate decreased thyroid function	About 5% of all patients develop goiters; evaluate triiodothyronine, thyroxine, and thyroid-stimulating hormone concentrations.
	Urine specific gravity	To detect diabetes insipidus	Specific gravity should be above 1.015.
Antipsychotics			
Acetophenazine	Blood counts	To detect blood dyscrasias	Phenothiazines can cause mild leukopenia; agranulocytosis is more frequently seen in females after 4 to 10 weeks of therapy. Incidence of blood dyscrasias is low but mortality is high; check blood studies promptly in symptomatic patients.
	Blood pressure	To detect adverse drug effects	Orthostatic hypotension may be problematic at initiation of therapy.
	ECG	To detect toxicity	Establish baseline and check periodically.
	Ophthalmologic examinations	To detect adverse drug effects	Corneal opacities and retinopathy have been reported after prolonged, high-dose therapy.

DRUG	TESTS	PURPOSE	SPECIAL CONSIDERATIONS
Antipsychotics *(continued)*			
Chlorproma-zine	Blood counts	To detect blood dyscrasias	Phenothiazines can cause mild leukopenia; agranulocytosis is more frequently seen in females after 4 to 10 weeks of therapy. Incidence of blood dyscrasias is low but mortality is high. Check blood studies promptly in symptomatic patients.
	Blood pressure	To detect adverse drug effects	Orthostatic hypotension may be problematic at initiation of therapy.
	ECG	To detect toxicity	Establish baseline and check periodically.
	Ophthalmologic exams	To detect adverse drug effects	Corneal opacities and retinopathy have been reported after prolonged, high-dose therapy.
Chlorprothix-ene	Blood counts	To detect blood dyscrasias	Drug can cause mild leukopenia or agranulocytosis. Incidence of blood dyscrasias is low. Check blood studies promptly in symptomatic patients.
	Blood pressure	To detect adverse drug effects	Orthostatic hypotension may be problematic at initiation of therapy.
	ECG	To detect toxicity	Establish baseline and repeat periodically.
	Ophthalmologic exams	To detect adverse drug effects	Corneal opacities and retinopathy may occur after prolonged, high-dose therapy.
Clozapine	Blood counts	To detect adverse drug effects	Drug can cause granulocytopenia or fatal agranulocytosis; baseline white blood cell (WBC) count and differential required before therapy, and weekly WBC and granulocyte counts are mandatory during therapy and for at least 4 weeks after drug is discontinued.

(continued)

DRUG	TESTS	PURPOSE	SPECIAL CONSIDERATIONS
Antipsychotics *(continued)*			
Droperidol	Blood counts	To detect blood dyscrasias	Drug can cause mild leukopenia or agranulocytosis. Incidence of blood dyscrasias is low. Check blood studies promptly in symptomatic patients.
	Blood pressure	To detect adverse drug effects	Orthostatic hypotension may be problematic at initiation of therapy; hypertension can occur with prolonged use.
	ECG	To detect toxicity	Establish baseline and repeat periodically.
Fluphen-azine	Blood counts	To detect blood dyscrasias	Phenothiazines can cause mild leukopenia; agranulocytosis is more common in females after 4 to 10 weeks of therapy. Incidence of blood dyscrasias is low but mortality is high. Check blood studies promptly in symptomatic patients.
	Blood pressure	To detect adverse drug effects	Orthostatic hypotension may be problematic at initiation of therapy.
	ECG	To detect toxicity	Establish baseline and repeat periodically.
	Ophthalmologic exams	To detect adverse drug effects	Corneal opacities and retinopathy have been reported after prolonged, high-dose therapy.
Haloperidol	Blood counts	To detect blood dyscrasias	Drug can cause mild leukopenia or agranulocytosis (only when combined with other drugs). Incidence of blood dyscrasias is low. Check blood studies promptly in symptomatic patients.
	Blood pressure	To detect adverse drug effects	Orthostatic hypotension may occur at start of therapy; hypertension can occur with prolonged use.
	ECG	To detect toxicity	Establish baseline and check periodically.

DRUG	TESTS	PURPOSE	SPECIAL CONSIDERATIONS
Antipsychotics *(continued)*			
Loxapine	Blood counts	To detect blood dyscrasias	Drug can cause mild leukopenia or agranulocytosis. Incidence of blood dyscrasias is low. Check blood studies promptly in symptomatic patients.
	Blood pressure	To detect adverse drug effects	Tachycardia or orthostatic hypotension may be problematic, especially at initiation of therapy.
	ECG	To detect toxicity	Establish baseline and repeat periodically.
	Ophthalmologic examinations	To detect adverse drug effects	Corneal opacities and retinopathy may occur after prolonged, high-dose therapy. Anticholinergic effects may aggravate glaucoma.
Mesoridazine	Blood counts	To detect blood dyscrasias	Phenothiazines can cause mild leukopenia; agranulocytosis is more common in females after 4 to 10 weeks of therapy. Incidence of blood dyscrasias is low but mortality is high. Check blood studies promptly in symptomatic patients.
	Blood pressure	To detect adverse drug effects	Orthostatic hypotension may be problematic at initiation of therapy.
	ECG	To detect toxicity	Establish baseline and repeat periodically.
	Ophthalmologic exams	To detect adverse drug effects	Corneal opacities and retinopathy have been reported after prolonged, high-dose therapy.
Molindone	Blood counts	To detect blood dyscrasias	Drug can cause mild leukopenia or agranulocytosis. Incidence of blood dyscrasias is low. Check blood studies promptly in symptomatic patients.
	Blood pressure	To detect adverse drug effects	Tachycardia or orthostatic hypotension may occur, especially at start of therapy.
	ECG	To detect toxicity	Establish baseline and repeat periodically.
	Ophthalmologic examinations	To detect adverse drug effects	Corneal opacities and retinopathy may occur after prolonged, high-dose therapy. Anticholinergic effects may aggravate glaucoma.

(continued)

DRUG	TESTS	PURPOSE	SPECIAL CONSIDERATIONS
Antipsychotics *(continued)*			
Perphena-zine	Blood counts	To detect blood dyscrasias	Drug can cause mild leukopenia; agranulocytosis is more common in females after 4 to 10 weeks of therapy. Incidence of blood dyscrasias is low but mortality is high. Check blood studies promptly in symptomatic patients.
	Blood pressure	To detect adverse drug effects	Orthostatic hypotension may occur at start of therapy.
	ECG	To detect toxicity	Establish baseline and repeat periodically.
	Ophthalmologic examinations	To detect adverse drug effects	Corneal opacities and retinopathy have been reported after prolonged, high-dose therapy.
Prochlorper-azine	Blood counts	To detect blood dyscrasias	Drug can cause mild leukopenia; agranulocytosis is more common in females after 4 to 10 weeks of therapy. Incidence of blood dyscrasias is low but mortality is high. Check blood studies promptly in symptomatic patients.
	Blood pressure	To detect adverse drug effects	Orthostatic hypotension may occur at start of therapy.
	ECG	To detect toxicity	Establish baseline and repeat periodically.
	Ophthalmologic examinations	To detect adverse drug effects	Corneal opacities and retinopathy have been reported after prolonged, high-dose therapy.
Promazine	Blood counts	To detect blood dyscrasias	Phenothiazines can cause mild leukopenia; agranulocytosis is more frequently seen in females after 4 to 10 weeks of therapy. Incidence of blood dyscrasias is low but mortality is high. Check blood studies promptly in symptomatic patients.
	Blood pressure	To detect adverse drug effects	Orthostatic hypotension may be problematic at initiation of therapy.
	ECG	To detect toxicity	Establish baseline and repeat periodically.
	Ophthalmologic examinations	To detect adverse drug effects	Corneal opacities and retinopathy have been reported after prolonged, high-dose therapy.

DRUG	TESTS	PURPOSE	SPECIAL CONSIDERATIONS
Antipsychotics *(continued)*			
Thioridazine	Blood counts	To detect blood dyscrasias	Phenothiazines can cause mild leukopenia; agranulocytosis is more frequently seen in females after 4 to 10 weeks of therapy. Incidence of blood dyscrasias is low but mortality is high. Check blood studies promptly in symptomatic patients.
	Blood pressure	To detect adverse drug effects	Orthostatic hypotension may be problematic at initiation of therapy.
	ECG	To detect toxicity	Establish baseline and repeat periodically.
	Ophthalmologic examinations	To detect adverse drug effects	Corneal opacities and retinopathy have been reported after prolonged, high-dose therapy.
Thiothixene	Blood counts	To detect blood dyscrasias	Drug can cause mild leukopenia or agranulocytosis. Incidence of blood dyscrasias is low. Check blood studies promptly in symptomatic patients.
	Blood pressure	To detect adverse drug effects	Orthostatic hypotension may be problematic at initiation of therapy.
	ECG	To detect toxicity	Establish baseline and repeat periodically.
	Ophthalmologic examinations	To detect adverse drug effects	Corneal opacities and retinopathy may occur after prolonged, high-dose therapy.
Trifluoperazine	Blood counts	To detect blood dyscrasias	Phenothiazines can cause mild leukopenia; agranulocytosis is more frequently seen in females after 4 to 10 weeks of therapy. Incidence of blood dyscrasias is low but mortality is high. Check blood studies promptly in symptomatic patients.
	Blood pressure	To detect adverse drug effects	Orthostatic hypotension may be problematic at initiation of therapy.
	ECG	To detect toxicity	Establish baseline and repeat periodically.
	Ophthalmologic examinations	To detect adverse drug effects	Corneal opacities and retinopathy have been reported after prolonged, high-dose therapy.

(continued)

DRUG	TESTS	PURPOSE	SPECIAL CONSIDERATIONS
Anxiolytics			
Alprazolam	Blood counts	To detect blood dyscrasias	Establish baseline and repeat periodically during prolonged therapy.
	Liver function tests	To detect hepatotoxicity	Elevated liver function tests reported after prolonged benzodiazepine use.
	Renal function tests	To detect nephrotoxicity	Decreased renal function may occur after prolonged benzodiazepine use.
Chlordiazepoxide	Blood counts	To detect blood dyscrasias	Establish baseline and repeat periodically during prolonged therapy.
	Liver function tests	To detect hepatotoxicity	Elevated liver function tests reported after prolonged benzodiazepine use.
	Renal function tests	To detect nephrotoxicity	Decreased renal function may occur after prolonged benzodiazepine use.
Diazepam	Blood counts	To detect blood dyscrasias	Relatively rare; establish baseline and repeat periodically during prolonged therapy.
	Liver function tests	To detect hepatotoxicity	Elevated aspartate aminotransferase, alanine aminotransferase, lactate dehydrogenase, alkaline phosphatase, and total and direct bilirubin levels reported occasionally with chronic use.
	Plasma testolactone levels	To detect chronic toxicity	Decreases reported in males with prolonged therapy.
	Renal function studies	To detect nephrotoxicity	May occur with prolonged use; also transient decreased renal function after parenteral diazepam has been reported.
Halazepam	Blood counts	To detect blood dyscrasias	Establish baseline and repeat periodically during prolonged therapy.
	Liver function tests	To detect hepatotoxicity	Elevated liver function tests reported after prolonged benzodiazepine use.
	Renal function tests	To detect nephrotoxicity	Decreased renal function may occur after prolonged benzodiazepine use.

DRUG	TESTS	PURPOSE	SPECIAL CONSIDERATIONS
Anxiolytics *(continued)*			
Lorazepam	Blood counts	To detect blood dyscrasias	Establish baseline and repeat periodically during prolonged use.
	Liver function tests	To detect hepatotoxicity	Elevated liver enzyme levels reported after prolonged benzodiazepine use.
	Renal function tests	To detect nephrotoxicity	Nephrotoxicity may occur after prolonged use.
Meprobamate	Blood counts	To detect blood dyscrasias	Establish baseline and repeat periodically; blood dyscrasias have been reported rarely.
Oxazepam	Blood counts	To detect blood dyscrasias	Establish baseline and repeat periodically.
	Liver function tests	To detect hepatotoxicity	May occur after prolonged benzodiazepine use.
	Renal function tests	To detect nephrotoxicity	May occur after prolonged benzodiazepine use.
Prazepam	Blood counts	To detect blood dyscrasias	Establish baseline and repeat periodically.
	Liver function tests	To detect hepatotoxicity	May occur after prolonged benzodiazepine use.
	Renal function tests	To detect nephrotoxicity	May occur after prolonged benzodiazepine use.
Sedative-hypnotics			
Amobarbital	Complete blood count (CBC), platelet count	To detect blood dyscrasias	Establish baseline and repeat periodically.
Aprobarbital	CBC, platelet count	To detect blood dyscrasias	Establish baseline and repeat periodically.
Butabarbital	CBC, platelet count	To detect blood dyscrasias	Establish baseline and repeat periodically.
Chloral hydrate	Blood counts	To detect blood dyscrasias	Leukopenia and eosinophilia reported rarely with prolonged use.

(continued)

DRUG	TESTS	PURPOSE	SPECIAL CONSIDERATIONS
Sedative-hypnotics *(continued)*			
Flurazepam	Blood counts	To detect blood dyscrasias	Establish baseline and repeat periodically.
	Liver function tests	To detect hepato-toxicity	Reported with prolonged benzodiazepine use.
	Renal function tests	To detect nephro-toxicity	Reported with prolonged benzodiazepine use.
Glutethimide	Blood counts	To detect blood dyscrasias	May be symptom of an acute hypersensitivity reaction.
Pentobarbital	CBC, platelet count	To detect blood dyscrasias	Establish baseline and repeat periodically.
Quazepam	Blood counts	To detect blood dyscrasias	Establish baseline and repeat periodically.
	Liver function tests	To detect hepato-toxicity	Reported with prolonged benzodiazepine use.
	Renal function tests	To detect nephro-toxicity	Reported with prolonged use of benzodiazepines.
Secobarbital	CBC, platelet count	To detect blood dyscrasias	Establish baseline and repeat periodically.
Temazepam	Blood counts	To detect blood dyscrasias	Establish baseline and repeat periodically.
	Liver function tests	To detect hepato-toxicity	Reported with prolonged benzodiazepine use.
	Renal function tests	To detect nephro-toxicity	Reported with prolonged benzodiazepine use.
Triazolam	Blood counts	To detect blood dyscrasias	Establish baseline and repeat periodically.
	Liver function tests	To detect hepato-toxicity	Reported with prolonged benzodiazepine use.
	Renal function tests	To detect nephro-toxicity	Reported with prolonged benzodiazepine use.

Drugs Associated with Psychiatric Symptoms

The following list identifies the generic names and pharmacologic classes of drugs that have been associated with psychiatric symptoms or disorders. The incidence of such reactions is presented as well.

SYMPTOM	GENERIC NAME	TRADE NAME	INCIDENCE
Agitation	alprazolam	Xanax	2.9%
	antidepressants		Common
	atropine sulfate		Common
	clonidine	Catapres	3%
	diphenhydramine	Benadryl	Less common
	ephedrine sulfate		Common
	fluoxetine	Prozac	Frequent
	indapamide	Lozol	5%
	monoamine oxidase (MAO) inhibitors		Frequent
	methadone hydrochloride	Dolophine	Less frequent
	morphine sulfate	Duramorph, MSIR	Less frequent
	paroxetine	Paxil	2.1%
	venlafaxine	Effexor	2%
Akathisia	alprazolam	Xanax	3%
	chlorprothixene	Taractan	Common
	phenothiazines		Common
Amnesia	alprazolam	Xanax	>1%
	benzodiazepines		Frequent in high doses
	triazolam	Halcion	0.5% to 0.9%
Anxiety	amantadine	Symmetrel	1% to 5%
	central nervous system (CNS) stimulants		Frequent
	diazoxide	Proglycem	Frequent
	dronabinol	Marinol	16%
	epinephrine	Adrenalin	Frequent
	indapamide	Lozol	5%
	indomethacin	Indocin	<1%
	leuprolide acetate	Lupron	>3%
	maprotiline	Ludiomil	3%
	naltrexone	Trexan	>7%
	oxymetazoline	Afrin, OcuClear	Frequent
	paroxetine	Paxil	5%
	pindolol	Visken	4%
	ritodrine	Yutopar	5% to 6% (I.V.)
	sympathomimetics		Frequent
	theophylline	Slo-Phyllin, Theolair	Common with overdose
	venlafaxine	Effexor	6%

(continued)

SYMPTOM	GENERIC NAME	TRADE NAME	INCIDENCE
Apathy	CNS depressants		Rare
	digitalis glycosides		Infrequent
	halazepam	Paxipam	9%
Behavioral	clonazepam	Klonopin	25%
changes	meperidine	Demerol	Common
Catatonia	beta-adrenergic blockers		Rare
	butyrophenones		Common
	methdilazine hydrochloride	Tacaryl	Uncommon
	perphenazine	Trilafon	Uncommon
	perphenazine and amitriptyline	Etrafon, Triavil	Uncommon
	phenothiazines		Uncommon
	prochlorperazine	Compazine	Uncommon
	promethazine	Phenergan	Uncommon
	thioxanthines		Uncommon
	trifluoperazine	Stelazine	Uncommon
	trimeprazine	Temaril	Uncommon
Choreoathe-	chlorprothixene	Taractan	Common
totic move-	levodopa	Larodopa	Frequent
ments	lithium	Cibalith, Eskalith, Lithane, Lithobid	Frequent with high lithium levels
	loxapine hydrochloride	Loxitane C	Infrequent
	methyldopa	Aldomet	Infrequent
	methyldopa and chlorothiazide	Aldoclor	Infrequent
	methyldopa and hydrochlorothiazide	Aldoril	Infrequent
Clonic move- ments	lithium	Cibalith, Eskalith, Lithane, Lithobid	Frequent with high lithium levels
Clonus	doxapram	Dopram	Rare
Confusion	alprazolam	Xanax	10.4%
	amantadine	Symmetrel	1% to 5%
	baclofen	Lioresal	1% to 11%
	benzodiazepines		Frequent
	bromocriptine	Parlodel	Common
	carbamazepine	Tegretol	Less frequent
	CNS depressants		Frequent
	cyclosporine	Sandimmune	2%
	diazepam	Valium	Infrequent
	esmolol	Brevibloc	2%
	guanadrel sulfate	Hylorel	14.8%
	halazepam	Paxipam	9%
	interferon alfa-2a, recombinant	Roferon-A	10%

SYMPTOM	GENERIC NAME	TRADE NAME	INCIDENCE
Confusion (continued)	isocarboxazid	Marplan	Most common
	levodopa	Larodopa	Frequent
	MAO inhibitors		Frequent
	metoclopramide	Octamide, Reglan	>10%
	mexiletine	Mexitil	2.6%
	paroxetine	Paxil	1.2%
	pentazocine	Talwin	30%
	phenobarbital		<1%
	phenytoin	Dilantin	Most common
	temazepam	Restoril	2% to 3%
	tocainide	Tonocard	>1%
	venlafaxine	Effexor	2%
Delirium	amphetamines		Infrequent
	anticholinergics		Frequent
	atropine sulfate		Frequent with toxic doses
	chloramphenicol	Chloromycetin	Infrequent
	cimetidine	Tagamet	Rare
	clonidine	Catapres	Rare
	corticosteroids		Infrequent
	ephedrine sulfate		Infrequent
	fentanyl citrate with droperidol	Innovar	Infrequent
	lorazepam	Ativan	Rare
	methohexital sodium	Brevital Sodium	Infrequent
	mexiletine	Mexitil	<1%
	opium alkaloids	Pantopon	Frequent
	phenelzine	Nardil	Rare
	phenylephrine	Neo-Synephrine	Rare
	phenylpropanolamine	Propagest	Frequent with overdose
	phenytoin	Dilantin	Frequent and dose-related
	quinidine gluconate	Quinaglute	Less frequent
	sympathomimetics		Frequent
	thiamylal	Surital	Frequent
Delusions	tricyclic antidepressants		Infrequent
	carbidopa-levodopa	Sinemet	<1%
	levodopa	Larodopa	Frequent
Dementia	carbidopa-levodopa	Sinemet	<1%
	levodopa	Larodopa	<1%
	quinidine sulfate	Quinidex Extentabs	Infrequent
Depression	alprazolam	Xanax	13.8%
	amantadine	Symmetrel	1% to 5%
	atenolol	Tenormin	12%
	atenolol and chlorthalidone	Tenoretic	12%
	baclofen	Lioresal	Rare
	clonidine	Catapres	1%
	dronabinol	Marinol	7%
	flecainide	Tambocor	1% to 3%
	flunisolide	Aerobid Inhaler	1% to 3%

(continued)

SYMPTOM	GENERIC NAME	TRADE NAME	INCIDENCE
Depression (continued)	guanabenz	Wytensin	3%
	guanadrel	Hylorel	1.9%
	halazepam	Paxipam	9%
	indapamide	Lozol	5%
	indomethacin	Indocin	1% to 3%
	metoclopramide	Octamide	<10%
	metoprolol	Lopressor	5%
	mexiletine	Mexitil	2.4%
	naltrexone	Trexan	<10%
	nonsteroidal anti-inflammatory drugs (NSAIDs)		<3%
	paroxetine	Paxil	1.2%
	pentazocine	Talwin	Infrequent
	ranitidine	Zantac	Rare
	reserpine	Serpasil	Frequent with high doses
	tolmetin	Tolectin	<3%
	triazolam	Halcion	0.5% to 0.9%
	venlafaxine	Effexor	1%
Disorientation	benzodiazepines		Frequent
	cimetidine	Tagamet	Rare
	CNS depressants		Frequent
	halazepam	Paxipam	9%
	lidocaine	Xylocaine	Less common
	meperidine	Demerol	Frequent
	methadone hydrochloride	Dolophine, Methadose	Less common
	metronidazole	Flagyl	<1%
	morphine	Duramorph, MSIR	Less frequent
	NSAIDs		<1%
	pentazocine	Talwin	30%
Dysphoria	metoclopramide	Octamide, Reglan	10%
	opiates		Frequent
Emotional disturbances	imipramine	Tofranil	Infrequent
	primidone	Mysoline	Less frequent
	ritodrine	Yulopar	5% to 6%
	valproic acid	Depakene	Frequent
Euphoria	antidepressants		Infrequent
	levodopa	Larodopa	Frequent
	methadone hydrochloride	Dolophine, Methadose	Less common
	morphine sulfate	Duramorph, MSIR	Less frequent
	pentazocine	Talwin	Frequent
Hallucinations	acyclovir	Zovirax	1%
	amantadine	Symmetrel	1% to 5%
	atropine sulfate		Frequent in toxic doses
	baclofen	Lioresal	Rare

SYMPTOM	GENERIC NAME	TRADE NAME	INCIDENCE
Hallucina-tions *(continued)*	beta-adrenergic blockers		Rare
	bromocriptine	Parlodel	Common
	carbidopa-levodopa	Sinemet	3.9%
	cimetidine	Tagamet	Rare
	corticosteroids		<1%
	diazepam	Valium	Rare
	digitalis glycosides		Rare
	dronabinol	Marinol	5%
	ephedrine sulfate	Ephed II	Infrequent
	famotidine	Pepcid	Infrequent
	levodopa	Larodopa	Frequent
	lidocaine	Xylocaine	Less common
	naltrexone	Trexan	<1%
	oxymetazoline	Afrin, OcuClear	Less frequent
	pentazocine	Talwin	Infrequent
	phenylephrine	Neo-Synephrine	Less frequent
	propranolol	Inderal	Infrequent
	ranitidine	Zantac	Rare
Hyperirrita-bility	dinoprostone	Prostin E$_2$	Infrequent
	phenylpropanolamine	Propagest	Common
	primidone	Mysoline	Less common
	thiabendazole	Mintezol	Frequent
Hysteria	azatidine	Optimine	Infrequent
	clemastine	Tavist	Infrequent
	clonazepam	Klonopin	Common
	cyproheptadine	Periactin	Infrequent
	dexchlorpheniramine, pseu-doephedrine, and guaifen-esin	Polaramine	Infrequent
	ethchlorvynol	Placidyl	Infrequent
	phenylpropanolamine and chlorpheniramine	Ornade, Triaminic	Frequent with high doses
	promethazine	Phenergan	Uncommon
	trimeprazine	Temaril	Uncommon
	tripelennamine	PBZ	Less frequent
	triprolidine, pseudoephed-rine, and codeine phos-phate	Actifed with co-deine	Infrequent
Insomnia	acebutolol	Sectral	3%
	albuterol	Proventil, Ventolin	2%
	alprazolam	Xanax	>8%
	amantadine	Symmetrel	5% to 10%
	amphetamines		Frequent
	antidepressants (selective serotonin reuptake inhibi-tors)		Common
	baclofen	Lioresal	2% to 7%
	clomiphene	Serophene	1.9%
	estramustine	Emcyt	3% to 4%

(continued)

SYMPTOM	GENERIC NAME	TRADE NAME	INCIDENCE
Insomnia (continued)	fluoxetine	Prozac	13.8%
	guanfacine	Tenex	4%
	indapamide	Lozol	<5%
	interferon alfa-2b, recombinant	Intron	5%
	isocarboxazid	Marplan	Most frequent
	ketoprofen	Orudis	>3%
	leuprolide acetate	Lupron	<3%
	MAO inhibitors		Common
	maprotiline	Ludiomil	2%
	metoclopramide	Octamide	10%
	pentoxifylline	Trental	2.3%
	phenylpropanolamine	Propagest	Frequent
	pindolol	Visken	19%
	sympathomimetics		Frequent
	theophylline	Slo-Phyllin, Theolair	Common
	venlafaxine	Effexor	18%
Irritability	amantadine	Symmetrel	1% to 5%
	dronabinol	Marinol	7%
	flunisolide	AeroBid Inhaler	3% to 9%
	indapamide	Lozol	5%
	naltrexone	Trexan	>10%
Jitteriness	acyclovir	Zovirax	1%
	amitriptyline	Elavil	Uncommon
	amphetamines		Frequent
	chlorpromazine	Thorazine	Frequent
	diethylpropion	Tenuate	Common
	isocarboxazid	Marplan	Most frequent
	metoclopramide	Octamide, Reglan	10%
	nifedipine	Adalat, Procardia	2%
	phenelzine	Nardil	Less frequent
	prochlorperazine	Compazine	Frequent
	ritodrine	Yutopar	5% to 8%
	sympathomimetics		Frequent
	trifluoperazine	Stelazine	Frequent
Lethargy	atenolol	Tenormin	3%
	atenolol and chlorthalidone	Tenoretic	3%
	butalbital, aspirin, caffeine and codeine phosphate	Fiorinal with codeine	Most common
	butorphanol	Stadol	2%
	clonidine	Catapres	3%
	estramustine	Emcyt	3% to 4%
	etretinate	Tegison	1% to 10%
	immune globulin	RhoGAM	25%
	indapamide	Lozol	5%
	interferon alfa-2a, recombinant	Roferon-A	3%
	leuprolide acetate	Lupron	3%
	metoprolol	Lopressor	10%
	pindolol	Visken	3%
	temazepam	Restoril	3%

SYMPTOM	GENERIC NAME	TRADE NAME	INCIDENCE
Manic symptoms	antidepressants		20% to 30%
	baclofen	Lioresal	Rare
	corticosteroids		<1%
	levodopa	Larodopa	Infrequent
	paroxetine	Paxil	1%
	triazolam	Halcion	Rare
Memory impairment	alprazolam	Xanax	>1%
	beta-adrenergic blockers		Rare
	benztropine	Cogentin	Frequent
	clonazepam	Klonopin	Frequent
	glutethimide	Doliden	<1%
	isocarboxazid	Marplan	Most frequent
	isoniazid (NH)	INH	Uncommon
	leuprolide acetate	Lupron	<3%
	lithium	Cibalith, Eskalith, Lithane, Lithobid	Uncommon but dose-dependent
	MAO inhibitors		Frequent
	maprotiline	Ludiomil	Rare
	oxazepam	Serax	Frequent
	phenobarbital	Barbita	>3%
	tocainide	Tonocard	<1%
	trazodone	Desyrel	>1%
	trizolam	Halcion	0.5% to 0.9%
Memory loss, short-term	benzodiazepines		Frequent
	mexiletine	Mexitil	<1%
	propranolol	Inderal	Infrequent
Mood changes	carbidopa-levodopa	Sinemet	2%
	fenfluramine	Pondimin	Frequent
	flunisolide	AeroBid Inhaler	1% to 3%
	hydrocodone and acetaminophen	Co-Gesic, Vicodin, Zydone	Less frequent
	hydrocodone, aspirin, and caffeine	Damason-P	Less frequent
	hydrocodone and chlorpheniramine	Hycomine	Less frequent
	hydromorphone	Dilaudid	Frequent
	methotrexate	Mexate	Rare
	nifedipine	Adalat, Procardia	7%
	piroxicam	Feldene	<1%
	tocainide	Tonocard	11%
Nervousness	albuterol	Proventil, Ventolin	4% to 20%
	alprazolam	Xanax	4.1%
	bitolterol	Tornalate	5%
	dicyclomine	Bentyl	6%
	flunisolide	AeroBid Inhaler	3% to 9%

(continued)

SYMPTOM	GENERIC NAME	TRADE NAME	INCIDENCE
Nervousness (continued)	indapamide	Lozol	>5%
	ipratropium bromide	Atrovent	3.1%
	isoetharine hydrochloride	Arm-a-Med Isoetharine	Common with excessive dosing
	ketoprofen	Orudis	>3%
	maprotiline	Ludiomil	6%
	metaproterenol	Alupent	14.1%
	mexiletine	Mexitil	5%
	naltrexone	Trexan	>10%
	nifedipine	Adalat, Procardia	7%
	paroxetine	Paxil	5.2%
	pindolol	Visken	11%
	ritodrine	Yutopar	5% to 6%
	tocainide	Tonocard	11.5%
	triazolam	Halcion	5.2%
	trihexyphenidyl	Artane	30% to 50%
	venlafaxine	Effexor	13%
Neuromuscular reactions, extrapyramidal	butyrophenones	Thorazine	Frequent
	chlorpromazine	Haldol	Frequent
	haloperidol		Frequent
	phenothiazines	Orap	Frequent
	pimozide	Compazine	Frequent
	prochlorperazine		Frequent
	thioxanthines	Stelazine	<1%
	trifluoperazine	Vincasar PFS	Frequent
	vincristine		Frequent
Nightmares	amoxapine	Asendin	>1%
	atropine sulfate		Infrequent
	beta-adrenergic blockers		<1%
	bromocriptine	Parlodel	Less common
	levodopa	Larodopa	Frequent
Night terrors	ethosuximide	Zarontin	Infrequent
Paradoxical anxiety	hydrochlorothiazide and deserpidine	Oreticyl	Infrequent
	perphenazine	Trilafon	Infrequent
Paranoia	alprazolam	Xanax	1.4%
	carbidopa-levodopa	Sinemet	<1%
	dronabinol	Marinol	2%
	indomethacin	Indocin	<1%
	lidocaine	Xylocaine	Less common
	meperidine	Demerol	<1%
	naltrexone	Trexan	<1%
	NSAIDs		<1%
	sympathomimetics		Infrequent
Parkinson-like symptoms	asparaginase	Elspar	Rare
	chlorothiazine and reserpine	Diupres	Rare
	chlorthalidone and reserpine	Demi-Regroton	Rare

SYMPTOM	GENERIC NAME	TRADE NAME	INCIDENCE
Parkinson-like symptoms *(continued)*	haloperidol	Haldol	Frequent
	hydrochlorothiazide and reserpine	Hydropres-25	Rare
	hydroflumethiazide	Saluron	Infrequent
	indomethacin	Indocin	<1%
	methychlothiazide and reserpine	Diutensen-R	Rare
	methyldopa	Aldomet	Infrequent
	methyldopa and chlorothiazine	Aldoclor	Infrequent
	methyldopa and hydrochlorothiazine	Aldoril	Infrequent
	metoclopramide	Octamide	0.2% to 2%
	metyrosine	Demser	10%
	phenothiazines		Common
	pimozide	Orap	Frequent
	polythiazide	Renese	Infrequent
	rauwolfia serpentina	Raudixin	Rare
	reserpine	Serpasil	Rare
	trichlormethiazide and reserpine	Metatensin	Rare
	trimethobenzamide	Tigan	Infrequent
Psychiatric disturbances	guanadrel	Hylorel	3.8%
	phenacemide	Phenurone	17%
Psychosis, activation	bromocriptine	Parlodel	<1%
	fluphenazine hydrochloride	Prolixin Hydrochloride	Infrequent
	perphenazine and amitriptyline	Erafon, Triavil	Infrequent
	prochlorperazine	Compazine	Infrequent
Psychosis, exacerbation	fluphenazine hydrochloride	Permetil Hydrochloride, Prolixin Hydrochloride	Infrequent
	thiethylperazine	Torecan	Infrequent
	thioridazine	Mellaril	Infrequent
	tricyclic antidepressants		Rare
Psychosis, toxic	isoniazid (INH)	INH	Uncommon
	methylphenidate	Ritalin	Uncommon
Psychosis	amantadine	Symmetrel	≤1%
	amphetamines		Rare
	bromocriptine	Parlodel	<1%
	chlorprothixene	Taractan	Infrequent
	cimetidine	Tagamet	Rare
	clonazepam	Klonopin	Infrequent

(continued)

SYMPTOM	GENERIC NAME	TRADE NAME	INCIDENCE
Psychosis *(continued)*	cycloserine	Seromycin	Infrequent, dose-dependent
	dapsone	Avlosulfon	Infrequent
	digoxin	Lanoxicaps, Lanoxin	1% to 4%
	divalproex sodium	Depakote	Infrequent
	hydroxychloroquine	Plaquenil	Infrequent
	Iohexol	Omnipaque	<1%
	methadone hydrochloride (I.V.)	Dolophine, Methadose	Rare
	methyldopa	Aldomet	Infrequent
	metrizamide	Amipaque	Rare
	phendimetrazine	Plegine	Rare
	phentermine	Adipex-P	Rare
	prednisolone sodium phosphate	Hydeltrasol	Infrequent
	procainamide	Pronestyl	Infrequent
	sulfisoxazole and phenazopyridine	Azo Gantrisin	Infrequent
	valproic acid	Depakene	Infrequent but dose-dependent
	vidarabine	Vira-A	Infrequent
Rage reactions	sulindac	Clinoril	1% to 3%
Seizures	alprazolam	Xanax	<1% (2 to 3 days after abrupt discontinuation)
	bromocriptine	Parlodel	Infrequent
	chloroquine	Aralen	Infrequent
	chlorpromazine	Thorazine	Infrequent
	cyclosporine	Sandimmune	>3%
	desipramine	Norpramin	Rare
	esmolol	Brevibloc	<1%
	fluphenazine	Permitil	Infrequent
	lithium	Cibalith-S, Eskalith, Lithane, Lithobid	Infrequent but dose-dependent
	methdilazine hydrochloride	Tacaryl	Infrequent
	methocarbamol	Robaxin	Infrequent
	metoclopramide	Octamide, Reglan	Rare
	metronidazole	Flagyl, Protostat	Less frequent
	mezlocillin	Mezlin	Rare, may be seen with anaphylactic reactions
	paramethadione	Paradione	Infrequent
	paroxetine	Paxil	0.1%
	pemoline	Cylert	<1%
	penicillin	Veetids, Beepen-VK	Rare, may be seen with anaphylactic reactions
	perphenazine	Etrafon, Triavil	Infrequent
	promethazine	Phenergan	Infrequent

SYMPTOM	GENERIC NAME	TRADE NAME	INCIDENCE
Seizures (continued)	ticarcillin/clavulanate	Timentin	Rare, may be seen with anaphylactic reactions
	tocainide	Tonocard	<1%
	trimeprazine	Temaril	Infrequent
	trimethadione	Tridione	Infrequent
Sensorium, clouded	beta-adrenergic blockers		Rare
	CNS depressants		<1%
Sleep disturbances	bromocriptine	Parlodel	<1%
	diazepam	Valium	Infrequent
	ethosuximide	Zarontin	Frequent
	guanabenz	Wytensin	3%
	guanadrel	Hylorel	2.1%
	imipramine	Tofranil	Frequent
	metoprolol	Lopressor	10%
	mexiletine	Mexitil	7.1%
	naltrexone	Trexan	>10%
	nifedipine	Adalat, Procardia	2%
Suicidal ideation	amitriptyline	Elavil	Rare
	carbidopa-levodopa	Sinemet	Rare
	chlorthalidone and reserpine	Demi-Regroton, Regroton	Rare
	clonazepam	Klonopin	Rare
	meprobamate	Meprospan, Miltown	Rare
Tardive dyskinesia	haloperidol	Haldol	Frequent
	loxapine hydrochloride	Loxitane C	Frequent
	metoclopramide	Octamide, Regian	<2%
	molindone	Moban	Rare
	phenothiazines		Frequent
	pimozide	Orap	Infrequent
Tourette syndrome	dextroamphetamine	Dexedrine	Infrequent
	methamphetamine	Desoxyn	Infrequent
	pemoline	Cylert	Infrequent
	methylphenidate	Ritalin	Rare

Schedules of Controlled Substances

The Drug Enforcement Administration (DEA) within the U.S. Department of Justice enforces the Controlled Substances Act of 1970, which regulates the manufacturing, distribution, and dispensing of drugs that have potential for abuse.

DEA schedules

The DEA divides drugs under its jurisdiction into five schedules based on their potential for abuse and physical and psychological dependence. Controlled substances are identified by schedule in the following list.

Schedule I (C-I): Drugs in this category have high abuse potential and no accepted medical use.

acetylmethadol
dihydromorphine
fenethylline
heroin
ketobemidone
LSD
marijuana

mescaline
methaqualone
methlyenedioxymethamphetamine (MDMA)
peyote
psilocybin
tetrahydrocannabinol
tilidine

Schedule II (C-II): Drugs in this category have high abuse potential associated with severe risk of dependence (opiates, amphetamines, barbiturates).

alfentanil hydrochloride
amobarbital
amobarbital sodium
amphetamine complex
amphetamine mixtures
amphetamine sulfate
cocaine
cocaine hydrochloride
codeine phosphate
codeine sulfate
dextroamphetamine sulfate
dihydrocodeine bitartrate
dronabinol
fentanyl citrate
fentanyl citrate and droperidol
hydrocodone bitartrate
hydromorphone hydrochloride
levomethadyl acetate hydrochloride

levorphanol tartrate
meperidine hydrochloride
methadone hydrochloride
methamphetamine hydrochloride
methylphenidate hydrochloride
morphine sulfate
opium tincture
oxycodone hydrochloride
oxycodone terephthalate
oxymorphone hydrochloride
pantopon (hydrochlorides of opium alkaloids)
pentobarbital
pentobarbital sodium
phenmetrazine hydrochloride
secobarbital
secobarbital sodium
sufentanil citrate

Schedule III (C-III): Drugs in this category have less abuse potential than schedule II drugs and a smaller risk of dependence (nonbarbiturate sedatives, nonamphetamine stimulants, limited amounts of certain opiates, and anabolic steroids).

aprobarbital
benzphetamine hydrochloride
butabarbital
butabarbital sodium
chlorphentermine hydrochloride
fluoxymesterone
glutethimide
methyltestosterone
methyprylon
nandrolone decanoate
nandrolone phenpropionate
oxymetholone

paregoric tincture
phendimetrazine
phendimetrazine tartrate
stanozolol
testolactone
testosterone
testosterone cypionate
testosterone enanthate
testosterone propionate
thiamylal sodium
thiopental sodium

Schedule IV (C-IV): Drugs in this category have less abuse potential than schedule III drugs and a limited risk of dependence (some sedative-hypnotics, anxiolytics, nonopiate analgesics, and central nervous system stimulants).

alprazolam
chloral hydrate
chlordiazepoxide
clonazepam
clorazepate dipotassium
diazepam
diethylpropion hydrochloride
estazolam
ethchlorvynol
fenfluramine hydrochloride
flurazepam hydrochloride
halazepam
lorazepam
mazindol
mephobarbital
meprobamate
methohexital sodium
oxazepam

paraldehyde
pemoline
pentazocine
phenobarbital
phenobarbital sodium
phentermine hydrochloride
prazepam
propoxyphene hydrochloride
propoxyphene hydrochloride and acetaminophen
propoxyphene hydrochloride and aspirin
propoxyphene napsylate
propoxyphene napsylate and acetaminophen
propoxyphene napsylate and aspirin
quazepam
temazepam
triazolam
zolpidem tartrate

Schedule V (C-V): Drugs in this category have limited abuse potential; they're primarily small amounts of opiates (codeine) used as antitussives or antidiarrheals. Under federal law, limited quantities of certain C-V drugs may be purchased without a prescription directly from a pharmacist. The purchaser must be at least age 18 and must furnish suitable identification. All such transactions must be recorded by the dispensing pharmacist.

ICD-9-CM Classification of Psychiatric Disorders

This appendix adapts the classification of mental disorders published in 1994 by the American Psychiatric Association in the *Diagnostic and Statistical Manual of Mental Disorders*, 4th edition *(DSM-IV)*. Beside most diagnostic labels, you'll find the related numerical code from the *International Classification of Diseases*, 9th revision, *Clinical Modification (ICD-9-CM)*. These codes standardize psychiatric diagnostic names and are used by insurance companies to determine reimbursement for psychiatric services.

In this appendix, you'll find these abbreviations:

NEC = not elsewhere classified
NOS = not otherwise specified
x (in diagnostic code) = specific code number required
... (ellipsis) = name of specific mental disorder or medical condition should be inserted. For example, *Delirium due to...* may become *Delirium due to hypothyroidism.*

ADJUSTMENT DISORDERS

309.xx Adjustment disorder
    .0 With depressed mood
    .24 With anxiety
    .28 With mixed anxiety and depressed mood
    .3 With disturbance of conduct
    .4 With mixed disturbance of emotions and conduct
    .9 Unspecified (Specify if acute or chronic.)

ANXIETY DISORDERS

293.89 Anxiety disorder due to...(Indicate the medical condition; specify if with generalized anxiety, panic attacks, or obsessive-compulsive symptoms.)
300.00 Anxiety disorder NOS
300.01 Panic disorder without agoraphobia
300.02 Generalized anxiety disorder
300.21 Panic disorder with agoraphobia
300.22 Agoraphobia without history of panic disorder
300.23 Social phobia (Specify if generalized.)
300.29 Specific phobia (Specify if animal, natural environment, blood-injection-injury, situational, or other type.)
300.3 Obsessive-compulsive disorder (Specify if with poor insight.)
308.3 Acute stress disorder
309.81 Posttraumatic stress disorder (Specify if acute, chronic, or with delayed onsets.)
Substance-induced anxiety disorder (Refer to substance-related disorders for substance-specific codes; specify if with generalized anxiety, panic attacks, obsessive-compulsive symptoms, or phobic symptoms; and specify if onset occurred during intoxication or during withdrawal.)

DELIRIUM, DEMENTIA, AND AMNESTIC AND OTHER COGNITIVE DISORDERS

Amnestic disorders
294.0 Amnestic disorder due to...
    (Indicate the medical condition; specify if transient or chronic.)
298.8 Amnestic disorder NOS
Substance-induced persisting amnestic disorder (Refer to substance-related disorders for substance-specific codes.)

Delirium
293.0 Delirium due to...(Indicate the medical condition.)
780.09 Delirium NOS
Delirium due to multiple etiologies (Code each of the specific etiologies.)
Substance intoxication delirium (Refer to substance-related disorders for substance-specific codes.)
Substance withdrawal delirium (Refer to substance-related disorders for substance-specific codes.)

Dementia
290.xx Dementia of the Alzheimer's type with early onset
.10 Uncomplicated
.11 With delirium
.12 With delusions
.13 With depressed mood (Specify if with behavioral disturbance.)
290.xx Dementia of the Alzheimer's type with late onset
.0 Uncomplicated
.3 With delirium
.20 With delusions
.21 With depressed mood (Specify if with behavioral disturbance.)
290.xx Vascular dementia
.40 Uncomplicated
.41 With delirium
.42 With delusions
.43 With depressed mood (Specify if with behavioral disturbance.)
290.10 Dementia due to Creutzfeldt-Jacob disease
290.10 Dementia due to Pick's disease
294.1 Dementia due to head trauma (also head injury)
294.1 Dementia due to Huntington's disease
294.1 Dementia due to Parkinson's disease
294.1 Dementia due to...(Indicate the medical condition not listed above.)
294.8 Dementia NOS
294.9 Dementia due to human immunodeficiency virus (HIV) disease (Also HIV infection affecting central nervous system)
Dementia due to multiple etiologies (Code each of the specific etiologies.)
Substance-induced persisting dementia (Refer to substance-related disorders for substance-specific codes.)

Other cognitive disorders
294.9 Cognitive disorder NOS

DISORDERS USUALLY FIRST DIAGNOSED IN INFANCY, CHILDHOOD, OR ADOLESCENCE

Attention-deficit and disruptive behavior disorders
312.8 Conduct disorder (Specify onset as childhood or adolescence.)
312.9 Disruptive behavior disorder NOS
313.81 Oppositional defiant disorder

314.xx Attention-deficit and hyperactivity disorder
.00 Predominantly inattentive type
.01 Combined type
.01 Predominantly hyperactive impulsive type
314.9 Attention-deficit and hyperactivity disorder NOS

Communication disorders
307.0 Stuttering
307.9 Communication disorder NOS
315.31 Expressive language disorder
315.31 Mixed receptive-expressive language disorder
315.39 Phonological disorder

Elimination disorders
307.6 Enuresis unrelated to a medical condition (Specify as nocturnal, diurnal, or nocturnal and diurnal.)
307.7 Encopresis without constipation and overflow incontinence
787.6 Encopresis with constipation and overflow incontinence

Feeding and eating disorders of infancy or early childhood
307.52 Pica
307.53 Rumination disorder
307.59 Feeding disorder of infancy or early childhood

Learning disorders
315.00 Reading disorder
315.1 Mathematics disorder
315.2 Disorder of written expression
315.9 Learning disorder NOS

Mental retardation
317 Mild retardation
318.0 Moderate retardation
318.1 Severe retardation
318.2 Profound retardation
319 Unspecified severity

Motor skills disorder
315.4 Developmental coordination disorder

Pervasive developmental disorders
299.00 Autistic disorder
299.10 Childhood disintegrative disorder
299.80 Asperger's disorder

299.80 Rett's disorder
299.80 Pervasive developmental disorder NOS

Tic disorders
307.20 Tic disorder NOS
307.21 Transient tic disorder (Specify as single episode or recurrent.)
307.22 Chronic motor or vocal tic disorder
307.23 Tourette disorder

Other disorders of infancy, childhood, or adolescence
307.3 Stereotypic movement disorder (Specify if with self-injurious behavior.)
309.21 Separation anxiety disorder (Specify if early onset.)
313.23 Selective mutism
313.89 Reactive attachment disorder of infancy or early childhood (Specify as inhibited or disinhibited.)
313.9 Disorder of infancy, childhood, or adolescence NOS

DISSOCIATIVE DISORDERS

300.12 Dissociative amnesia
300.13 Dissociative fugue
300.14 Dissociative identity disorder
300.15 Dissociative disorder NOS
300.6 Depersonalization disorder

EATING DISORDERS
307.1 Anorexia nervosa (Specify if restricting type or binge-eating and purging type.)
307.50 Eating disorder NOS
307.51 Bulimia nervosa (Specify if purging or nonpurging type.)

FACTITIOUS DISORDERS

300.xx Factitious disorder
  .16 With predominantly psychological signs and symptoms
  .19 With predominantly physical signs and symptoms
  .19 With combined psychological and physical signs and symptoms
300.19 Factitious disorder NOS

IMPULSE-CONTROL DISORDERS NEC

312.30 Impulse-control disorder NOS
312.31 Pathological gambling
312.32 Kleptomania
312.33 Pyromania
312.34 Intermittent explosive disorder
312.39 Trichotillomania

MENTAL DISORDERS DUE TO A MEDICAL CONDITION NEC

293.89 Catatonic disorder due to...(Indicate the medical condition.)
293.9 Mental disorder NOS due to...(Indicate the medical condition.)
310.1 Personality change due to...(Indicate the medical condition; specify type: labile, disinhibited, aggressive, apathetic, paranoid, other, combined, or unspecified.)

MOOD DISORDERS

Bipolar disorders
293.83 Mood disorder due to...(Indicate the medical condition; specify if with depressive features, with major depressive-like episode, with manic features, or with mixed features.)
296.xx Bipolar I disorder
  .0x Single manic episode (Specify if mixed.)
  .40 Most recent episode hypomanic
  .4x Most recent episode manic
  .5x Most recent episode depressed
  .6x Most recent episode mixed
  .7 Most recent episode unspecified
296.89 Bipolar II disorder (Specify current or most recent episode as hypomanic or depressed.)
296.80 Bipolar disorder NOS
296.90 Mood disorder NOS
301.13 Cyclothymic disorder
Substance-induced mood disorder (Refer to substance-related disorders for substance-specific codes; specify if with depressive features, with manic features, or with mixed features; also

specify if onset occurred during intoxication or during withdrawal.)

Depressive disorders
296.xx Major depressive disorder
  .2x Single episode
  .3x Recurrent
300.4 Dysthymic disorder (Specify if early or late onset and if with atypical features.)
311 Depressive disorder NOS

PERSONALITY DISORDERS

301.0 Paranoid personality disorder
301.4 Obsessive-compulsive personality disorder
301.6 Dependent personality disorder
301.7 Antisocial personality disorder
301.20 Schizoid personality disorder
301.22 Schizotypal personality disorder
301.50 Histrionic personality disorder
301.81 Narcissistic personality disorder
301.82 Avoidant personality disorder
301.83 Borderline personality disorder
301.9 Personality disorder NOS

SCHIZOPHRENIA AND OTHER PSYCHOTIC DISORDERS

95.xx Schizophrenia
  The following classification applies to all subtypes of schizophrenia: episodic with interepisode residual symptoms (specify if with prominent negative symptoms), episodic with no interepisode residual symptoms, continuous (specify if with prominent negative symptoms), single episode in partial remission (specify if with prominent negative symptoms or single episode in full remission), or other or unspecified pattern.
  .10 Disorganized type
  .20 Catatonic type
  .30 Paranoid type
  .60 Residual type
  .90 Undifferentiated type
293.xx Psychotic disorder due to...(Indicate the medical condition.)
  .81 With delusions
  .82 With hallucinations
Substance-induced psychotic disorder (Refer to substance-related disorders

for substance-specific codes; specify with onset during intoxication or during withdrawal.)
295.40 Schizophreniform disorder (Specify with or without good prognostic features.)
295.70 Schizoaffective disorder (Specify bipolar or depressive type.)
297.1 Delusional disorder (Specify erotomanic, grandiose, jealous, persecutory, somatic, mixed, or unspecified type.)
297.3 Shared psychotic disorder
298.8 Brief psychotic disorder (Specify with or without marked stressors, or with postpartum onset.)
298.9 Psychotic disorder NOS

SEXUAL AND GENDER IDENTITY DISORDERS

Gender identity disorders
302.xx Gender identity disorder
  .6 In children
  .8 In adolescents or adults (Specify if sexually attracted to males, females, both, or neither.)
302.6 Gender identity disorder NOS

Paraphilias
302.2 Pedophilia (Specify if sexually attracted to males, females, or both; specify if limited to incest; and specify if exclusive or nonexclusive type.)
302.3 Transvestic fetishism (Specify if with gender dysphoria.)
302.4 Exhibitionism
302.81 Fetishism
302.82 Voyeurism
302.83 Sexual masochism
302.84 Sexual sadism
302.89 Frotteurism
302.9 Paraphilia NOS

Sexual dysfunctions
For all primary sexual dysfunctions, specify if lifelong or acquired type, generalized or situational type, and whether due to psychological factors or combined factors.

Orgasmic disorders
302.73 Female orgasmic disorder
302.74 Male orgasmic disorder
302.75 Premature ejaculation

Sexual arousal disorders
302.72 Female sexual arousal disorder
302.72 Male erectile disorder

Sexual desire disorders
302.71 Hypoactive sexual desire disorder
302.79 Sexual aversion disorder

Sexual dysfunction due to a medical condition
302.70 Sexual dysfunction NOS
607.84 Male erectile disorder due to...(Indicate the medical condition.)
608.89 Male dyspareunia due to...(Indicate the medical condition.)
608.89 Male hypoactive sexual desire disorder due to...(Indicate the medical condition.)
608.89 Other male sexual dysfunction due to...(Indicate the medical condition.)
Substance-induced sexual dysfunction (Refer to substance-related disorders for substance-specific codes; specify if with impaired desire, with impaired arousal, with impaired orgasm, or with sexual pain; and specify if onset occurred during intoxication.)
625.0 Female dyspareunia due to...(Indicate the medical condition.)
625.8 Female hypoactive sexual desire disorder due to...(Indicate the medical condition.)
625.8 Other female sexual dysfunction due to...(Indicate the medical condition.)

Sexual pain disorders
302.76 Dyspareunia (not due to a medical condition)
306.51 Vaginismus (not due to a medical condition)

Other sexual disorders
302.9 Sexual disorder NOS

SLEEP DISORDERS

Primary sleep disorders
Dyssomnias
307.42 Primary insomnia

307.44 Primary hypersomnia (Specify if recurrent.)
307.45 Circadian rhythm sleep disorder (Specify if delayed sleep phase, jet lag, shift work, or unspecified type.)
307.47 Dyssomnia NOS
347 Narcolepsy
80.59 Breathing-related sleep disorder

Parasomnias
307.46 Sleep terror disorder
307.46 Sleeping walking disorder
307.47 Nightmare disorder
307.47 Parasomnia NOS

Sleep disorders related to another mental disorder
307.42 Insomnia related to...(Indicate the disorder.)
307.44 Hypersomnia related to...(Indicate the disorder.)

Other sleep disorders
780.xx Sleep disorder due to...(Indicate the medical condition.)
  .52 Insomnia type
  .54 Hypersomnia type
  .59 Mixed type
  .59 Parasomnia type
Substance-induced sleep disorder (Refer to substance-related disorders for substance-specific codes; specify if insomnia, hypersomnia, parasomnia, or mixed type; and specify if onset occurred during intoxication or withdrawal.)

SOMATOFORM DISORDERS

300.7 Body dysmorphic disorder
300.7 Hypochondriasis (Specify if with poor insight.)
300.11 Conversion disorder (Specify if with motor symptom or deficit, sensory symptom or deficit, seizures or convulsions, or mixed presentation.)
300.81 Somatization disorder
300.81 Undifferentiated somatoform disorder
300.81 Somatoform disorder NOS
307.xx Pain disorder
  .80 Associated with psychological factors

.89 Associated with both psychological factors and a medical condition (Specify if acute or chronic.)

SUBSTANCE-RELATED DISORDERS

Alcohol-related disorders
Alcohol-induced disorders
291.0 Alcohol intoxication delirium
291.0 Alcohol withdrawal delirium
291.1 Alcohol-induced persisting amnestic disorder
291.2 Alcohol-induced persisting dementia
291.x Alcohol-induced psychotic disorder
   .3 With hallucinations (Specify if onset occurred during intoxication or withdrawal.)
   .5 With delusions (Specify if onset occurred during intoxication or withdrawal.)
291.8 Alcohol-induced anxiety disorder (Specify if onset occurred during intoxication or withdrawal.)
291.8 Alcohol-induced mood disorder (Specify if onset occurred during intoxication or withdrawal.)
291.8 Alcohol-induced sexual dysfunction (Specify with onset during intoxication.)
291.8 Alcohol withdrawal (Specify if with perceptual disturbances.)
291.9 Alcohol-induced sleep disorder (Specify if onset occurred during intoxication or withdrawal.)
291.9 Alcohol-related disorder NOS
303.00 Alcohol intoxication

Alcohol use disorders
303.90 Alcohol dependence (Specify with or without physiological dependence.)
305.00 Alcohol abuse

Amphetamine-related disorders
Amphetamine-induced disorders
292.0 Amphetamine withdrawal
292.xx Amphetamine-induced psychotic disorder
   .11 With delusions (Specify if onset occurred during intoxication.)
   .12 With hallucinations (Specify if onset occurred during intoxication.)
292.81 Amphetamine intoxication delirium

292.84 Amphetamine-induced mood disorder (Specify if onset occurred during intoxication or withdrawal.)
292.89 Amphetamine-induced anxiety disorder (Specify if onset occurred during intoxication.)
292.89 Amphetamine-induced sexual dysfunction (Specify if onset occurred during intoxication.)
292.89 Amphetamine-induced sleep disorder (Specify if onset occurred during intoxication or withdrawal.)
292.89 Amphetamine intoxication (Specify if with perceptual disturbances.)
292.9 Amphetamine-related disorder NOS

Amphetamine use disorders
304.40 Amphetamine dependence (Specify with or without physiological dependence.)
305.70 Amphetamine abuse

Caffeine-related disorders
Caffeine-induced disorders
292.89 Caffeine-induced anxiety disorder (Specify if onset occurred during intoxication.)
292.89 Caffeine-induced sleep disorder (Specify if onset occurred during intoxication.)
292.9 Caffeine-related disorder NOS
305.90 Caffeine intoxication

Cannabis-related disorders
Cannabis-induced disorders
292.xx Cannabis-induced psychotic disorder
   .11 With delusions (Specify if onset occurred during intoxication.)
   .12 With hallucinations (Specify if onset occurred during intoxication.)
292.81 Cannabis intoxication delirium
292.89 Cannabis-induced anxiety disorder (Specify if onset occurred during intoxication.)
292.89 Cannabis intoxication (Specify if with perceptual disturbances.)
292.9 Cannabis-related disorder NOS

Cannabis use disorders
304.30 Cannabis dependence (Specify with or without physiologic dependence.)
305.20 Cannabis abuse

Cocaine-related disorders
Cocaine-induced disorders
292.0 Cocaine withdrawal
292.xx Cocaine-induced psychotic disorders
  .11 With delusions (Specify if onset occurred during intoxication.)
  .12 With hallucinations (Specify if onset occurred during intoxication.)
292.81 Cocaine intoxication delirium
292.84 Cocaine-induced mood disorder (Specify if onset occurred during intoxication or withdrawal.)
292.89 Cocaine-induced anxiety disorder (Specify if onset occurred during intoxication or withdrawal.)
292.89 Cocaine-induced sexual dysfunction (Specify if onset occurred during intoxication.)
292.89 Cocaine-induced sleep disorder (Specify if onset occurred during intoxication or withdrawal.)
292.89 Cocaine intoxication (Specify if with perceptual disturbances.)
292.9 Cocaine-related disorder NOS

Cocaine use disorders
304.20 Cocaine dependence (Specify with or without physiologic dependence.)
305.60 Cocaine abuse

Hallucinogen-related disorders
Hallucinogen-induced disorders
292.xx Hallucinogen-induced psychotic disorder
  .11 With delusions (Specify if onset occurred during intoxication.)
  .12 With hallucinations (Specify if onset occurred during intoxication.)
292.81 Hallucinogen intoxication delirium
292.84 Hallucinogen-induced mood disorder (Specify if onset occurred during intoxication.)
292.89 Hallucinogen-induced anxiety disorder (Specify if onset occurred during intoxication.)
292.89 Hallucinogen intoxication
292.89 Hallucinogen persisting perception disorder (flashbacks)
292.9 Hallucinogen-related disorder NOS

Hallucinogen use disorders
304.50 Hallucinogen dependence (Specify with or without physiologic dependence.)

305.30 Hallucinogen abuse

Inhalant-related disorders
Inhalant-induced disorders
292.xx Inhalant-induced psychotic disorder
  .11 With delusions (Specify if onset occurred during intoxication.)
  .12 With hallucinations (Specify if onset occurred during intoxication.)
292.81 Inhalant intoxication delirium
292.82 Inhalant-induced persisting dementia
292.84 Inhalant-induced mood disorder (Specify if onset occurred during intoxication.)
292.89 Inhalant-induced anxiety disorder (Specify if onset occurred during intoxication.)
292.89 Inhalant intoxication
292.9 Inhalant-related disorder NOS

Inhalant use disorders
304.60 Inhalant dependence (Specify with or without physiologic dependence.)
305.90 Inhalant abuse

Nicotine-related disorders
Nicotine-induced disorders
292.0 Nicotine withdrawal
292.9 Nicotine-related disorder NOS

Nicotine use disorder
305.10 Nicotine dependence (Specify with or without physiologic dependence.)

Opioid-related disorders
Opioid-induced disorders
292.0 Opioid withdrawal
292.xx Opioid-induced psychotic disorder
  .11 With delusions (Specify if onset occurred during intoxication.)
  .12 With hallucinations (Specify if onset occurred during intoxication.)
292.81 Opioid intoxication delirium
292.84 Opioid-induced mood disorder (Specify if onset occurred during intoxication.)
292.89 Opioid-induced sexual dysfunction (Specify if onset occurred during intoxication.)
292.89 Opioid-induced sleep disorder (Specify if onset occurred during intoxication or withdrawal.)

292.89 Opioid intoxication (Specify if with perceptual disturbances.)
292.9 Opioid-related disorder NOS

Opioid use disorders
304.00 Opioid dependence (Specify with or without physiologic dependence.)
305.50 Opioid abuse

Phencyclidine-related disorders
Phencyclidine-induced disorders
292.xx Phencyclidine-induced psychotic disorder
  .11 With delusions (Specify if onset occurred during intoxication.)
  .12 With hallucinations (Specify if onset occurred during intoxication.)
292.81 Phencyclidine intoxication delirium
292.84 Phencyclidine-induced mood disorders (Specify if onset occurred during intoxication.)
292.89 Phencyclidine-induced anxiety disorders (Specify if onset occurred during intoxication.)
292.89 Phencyclidine intoxication (Specify if with perceptual disturbances.)
292.9 Phencyclidine-related disorder NOS

Phencyclidine use disorders
304.90 Phencyclidine dependence (Specify with or without physiologic dependence.)
305.90 Phencyclidine abuse

Polysubstance-related disorder
304.80 Polysubstance dependence (Specify with or without physiologic dependence.)

Sedative-, hypnotic-, or anxiolytic-related disorders
Sedative-, hypnotic-, or anxiolytic-induced disorders
292.0 Sedative, hypnotic, or anxiolytic withdrawal (Specify if with perceptual disturbances.)
292.xx Sedative-, hypnotic-, or anxiolytic-induced psychotic disorder
  .11 With delusions (Specify if onset occurred during intoxication.)
  .12 With hallucinations (Specify if onset occurred during intoxication.)
292.81 Sedative, hypnotic, or anxiolytic intoxication delirium

292.81 Sedative, hypnotic, or anxiolytic withdrawal delirium
292.82 Sedative-, hypnotic-, or anxiolytic-induced persisting dementia
292.83 Sedative-, hypnotic-, or anxiolytic-induced persisting amnestic disorder
292.84 Sedative-, hypnotic-, or anxiolytic-induced mood disorder (Specify if onset occurred during intoxication or withdrawal.)
292.89 Sedative-, hypnotic-, or anxiolytic-induced anxiety disorder (Specify if onset occurred during intoxication or withdrawal.)
292.89 Sedative-, hypnotic-, or anxiolytic-induced sexual dysfunction (Specify if onset occurred during intoxication.)
292.89 Sedative-, hypnotic-, or anxiolytic-induced sleep disorder (Specify if onset occurred during intoxication or withdrawal.)
292.89 Sedative, hypnotic, or anxiolytic intoxication
292.9 Sedative-, hypnotic-, or anxiolytic-related disorder NOS

Sedative, hypnotic, or anxiolytic use disorders
304.10 Sedative, hypnotic, or anxiolytic dependence (Specify with or without physiologic dependence.)
305.40 Sedative, hypnotic, or anxiolytic abuse

Other (or unknown) substance-related disorders
Other (or unknown) substance-induced disorders
292.0 Other (or unknown) substance withdrawal (Specify if with perceptual disturbances.)
292.xx Other (or unknown) substance-induced psychotic disorder
  .11 With delusions (Specify if onset occurred during intoxication.)
  .12 With hallucinations (Specify if onset occurred during intoxication.)
292.81 Other (or unknown) substance-induced delirium
292.82 Other (or unknown) substance-induced persisting dementia
292.83 Other (or unknown) substance-induced persisting amnestic disorder

292.84 Other (or unknown) substance-induced mood disorder (Specify if onset occurred during intoxication.)

292.89 Other (or unknown) substance-induced anxiety disorder (Specify if onset occurred during intoxication.)

292.89 Other (or unknown) substance-induced sexual dysfunction (Specify if onset occurred during intoxication.)

292.89 Other (or unknown) substance-induced sleep disorder (Specify if onset occurred during intoxication.)

292.89 Other (or unknown) substance intoxication (Specify if with perceptual disturbances.)

292.9 Other (or unknown) substance-related disorder NOS

Other (or unknown) substance use disorders

304.90 Other (or unknown) substance dependence (Specify with or without physiologic dependence.)

305.90 Other (or unknown) substance abuse

OTHER CONDITIONS

Abuse or neglect

V61.1 Physical abuse of adult (Code **995.81** if focus is on victim.)

V61.1 Sexual abuse of adult (Code **995.81** if focus is on victim.)

V61.21 Neglect of child (Code **995.5** if focus is on victim.)

V61.21 Physical abuse of child (Code **995.5** if focus is on victim.)

V61.21 Sexual abuse of child (Code **995.5** if focus is on victim.)

Medication-induced movement disorders

332.1 Neuroleptic-induced parkinsonism

333.1 Medication-induced postural tremor

333.7 Neuroleptic-induced acute dystonia

333.82 Neuroleptic-induced tardive dyskinesia

333.90 Medication-induced movement disorder NOS

333.92 Neuroleptic malignant syndrome

333.99 Neuroleptic-induced acute akathisia

Other medication-induced disorder

995.2 Adverse effects of medication NOS

Psychological factors affecting medical condition

316 Specified psychological factor affecting...(Indicate the medical condition.) Choose name based on nature of mental disorder, psychological symptoms, personality traits or coping style, maladaptive health behaviors, stress-related physiological response, and other factors that affect medical condition.

Relational problems

V61.1 Partner relational problem

V61.20 Parent-child relational problem

V61.8 Sibling relational problem

V62.81 Relational problem NOS

V61.9 Relational problem related to a mental disorder or medical condition

Additional conditions

313.82 Identity problem

780.9 Age-related cognitive decline

V15.81 Noncompliance with treatment

V62.2 Occupational problem

V62.3 Academic problem

V62.4 Acculturation problem

V62.82 Bereavement

V62.89 Borderline intellectual functioning

V62.89 Phase of life problem

V62.89 Religious or spiritual problem

V65.2 Malingering

V71.01 Adult antisocial behavior

V71.02 Child or adolescent antisocial behavior

Index

i refers to an illustration; t refers to a table

i refers to an illustration; t refers to a table

i refers to an illustration; t refers to a table

i refers to an illustration; t refers to a table

i refers to an illustration; t refers to a table

i refers to an illustration; t refers to a table

i refers to an illustration; t refers to a table